P9-AQF-158

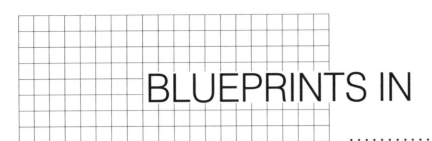

BLUEPRINTS IN

SURGERY

Seth J. Karp, MD
Resident in Surgery
Brigham and Women's Hospital
Clinical Fellow
Harvard Medical School
Boston, Massachusetts

James Morris, MD
Clinical Fellow
Harvard Medical School
Resident in Surgery
Massachusetts General Hospital
Boston, Massachusetts

Faculty Advisor:
David Soybel, MD
Assistant Professor of Surgery
Harvard Medical School
Division of General/Gastrointestinal Surgery
Brigham and Women's Hospital
Boston, Massachusetts

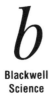

**Blackwell
Science**

Blackwell Science

Editorial Offices:
350 Main Street, Malden, Massachusetts 02148, USA
Osney Mead, Oxford OX2 0El, England
25 John Street, London WC1N 2BL, England
23 Ainslie Place, Edinburgh EH3 6AJ, Scotland
54 University Street, Carlton, Victoria 3053, Australia

Other Editorial Offices:
Arnette Blackwell SA, 224, Boulevard Saint Germain, 75007 Paris, France
Blackwell Wissenschafts-Verlag GmbH Kurfürstendamm 57, 10707 Berlin, Germany
Zehetnergasse 6, A-1140 Vienna, Austria

Distributors:

USA
Blackwell Science, Inc.
Commerce Place
350 Main Street
Malden, Massachusetts 02148
(Telephone orders: 800-215-1000
or 617-388-8250; Fax orders: 617-388-8270)

Canada
Copp Clark Professional
200 Adelaide Street, West, 3rd Floor
Toronto, Ontario M5H 1W7
(Telephone orders: 416-597-1616
or 1-800-815-9417; Fax orders: 416-597-1617)

Australia
Blackwell Science Pty., Ltd.
54 University Street
Carlton, Victoria 3053
(Telephone orders: 03-9347-0300;
Fax orders: 03-9349-3016)

Outside North America and Australia
Blackwell Science, Ltd.
c/o Marston Book Services, Ltd.
P.O. Box 269, Abingdon
Oxon OX14 4YN
England
(Telephone orders: 44-01235-465500;
Fax orders: 44-01235-465555)

Acquisitions: Joy Ferris Denomme
Production: Karen Feeney
Manufacturing: Lisa Flanagan
Typeset by Publication Services
Printed and bound by Capital City Press
© 1998 by Blackwell Science, Inc.
Printed in the United States of America

98 99 00 5 4 3 2 1

All rights reserved. No part of this book may be reproduced in any form or by any electronic or mechanical means, including information storage and retrieval systems, without permission in writing from the publisher, except by a reviewer who may quote brief passages in a review.

The Blackwell Science logo is a trade mark of Blackwell Science Ltd., registered at the United Kingdom Trade Marks Registry

Library of Congress Cataloging-in-Publication Data
Karp, Seth J.
    Blueprints in surgery / by Seth J. Karp, James Morris; Faculty Advisor, David
Soybel.
        p.   cm.—(The blueprints series)
    Includes bibliographical references and index.
    ISBN 0-86342-348-9
    1. Surgery—Outlines, syllabi, stc. I. Morris, James, 1964—
II. Title. III. Series.
    [DALM: 1. Surgery, Operative.   WO 500 K18p 1997]
RD37.3.K37   1997
617'.91—dc21
DNLM/DLC
For Library of Congress   97-7348
                                                        CIP

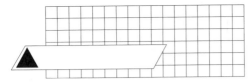

Contents

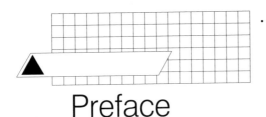

Preface

*F*ourth-year medical students, interns, and residents are chronically sleep deprived, have little time to study due to their clinical duties, and have a low tolerance for medical literature that is not clear and to the point. All too often as a medical student, and now as a resident, I have heard my colleagues bemoan the fact that there is no succinct, clinical text on each of the core subjects tested on the USMLE Steps 2 & 3. These trainees need review materials they can digest quickly, perhaps a subject in a weekend, which will enable them to answer correctly the majority of questions in each discipline. This attitude is especially evident for the USMLE Step 3 for example, where surgical residents are tested on pediatrics although they have not completed a clinical rotation in the discipline for two years.

Our goal in writing *Blueprints in Surgery* was to enable the reader to review the core material quickly and efficiently. The topics were chosen after analyzing over 2,000 review questions, which we believed were representative of the surgery questions on the USMLE Steps 2 & 3 exams. This book is not meant to be comprehensive, but rather it is composed of the "high-yield" topics that consistently appear on these exams.

The questions on the USMLE Steps 2 & 3 are now crafted into clinical vignettes. To assist you in studying for this new format, the material in this book is presented either as the workup of a symptom or as a discussion of a particular disease or pathological process. Although this series is designed for the medical student or resident reviewing for the USMLE, we believe the books will be equally useful to all medical students during their clerkships or subinternships.

We hope that you find *Blueprints in Surgery* informative and useful. We welcome any feedback you may have about this text or any others in the Blueprints series. Please feel free to send us your comments and suggestions and we will send you a free copy of any one of the Blueprints' books!

Bradley S. Marino, MD, MPP
Blueprints Series Editor
c/o Blackwell Science, Inc.
Commerce Place
350 Main Street
Malden, MA 02148

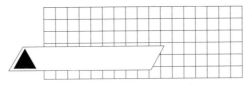

Acknowledgments

To the residents of the Department of Surgery at the Brigham and Women's Hospital and West Roxbury V.A.M.C. and to the Harvard and visiting medical students who have taught us all.

D.S.

To Sarah—S.K.

To Caroline—J.M.

Figure Credits

The following figures were modified with permission from the publisher.

Fig. 13-1. Lyons MK, Meyer FB. Cerebrospinal fluid physiology and the management of increased intracranial pressure. Mayo Clin Proc 1990;65:687.

Fig. 13-2. Fishman RA. Brain edema. N Engl J Med 1975; 293:706.

Fig. 13-3. Anderson J. Grant's Atlas of Anatomy. 8th ed. Baltimore: Williams & Wilkins, 1983.

Fig. 13-4. Dimsdale H, Logue V. Ruptured posterior fossa aneurysms and their surgical treatment. J Neurol Neurosurg Psychiatry 1959;22:202-217.

Fig. 13-5. Hosp. Med. 1965;1:9.

Fig. 13-6. Hosp. Med. 1965;1:9.

Fig. 13-7. Burger PC, Scheithaver BW, Vogel FS. Surgical pathology of the nervous system and its covering. 3rd ed. New York: Churchill Livingstone, 1991.

Fig. 13-8. Anderson J. Grant's Atlas of Anatomy. 8th ed. Baltimore: Williams & Wilkins, 1983.

Fig. 13-9. Morris PJ, Malt RA. Oxford Textbook of Surgery. Oxford: Oxford University Press, 1994:2184

Fig. 13-10. Morris PJ, Malt RA, Oxford Textbook of Surgery. Oxford: Oxford University Press, 1994:2187.

Fig. 15-1. Sabiston DC. Textbook of Surgery. The biological basis of modern surgical practice. 14th ed. Philadelphia: Saunders, 1991:1077.

Fig. 15-2. Lawrence PF. Essentials of General Surgery. Baltimore: Williams & Wilkins, 1988:246.

Fig. 15-3. Lawrence PF. Essentials of General Surgery. Baltimore: Williams & Wilkins, 1988:246.

Fig. 15-4. Lawrence PF. Essentials of General Surgery. Baltimore: Williams & Wilkins, 1988:247.

Fig. 15-5. Sabiston DC. Textbook of Surgery. The biological basis of modern surgical practice. 14th ed. Philadelphia: Saunders, 1991:1078.

Fig. 15-6. Simmons RL, Steed DL. Basic Science Review for Surgeons. Philadelphia: Saunders, 1992:263.

Fig. 15-7. Morris PJ, Malt RA, Oxford Textbook of Surgery. Oxford: Oxford University Press, 1994:1304.

Fig. 15-8. Way LW. Current Surgical Diagnosis and Treatment. 9th ed. Norwalk, CT: Appleton & Lange, 1991:578.

Fig. 16-1. Sabiston DC. Textbook of Surgery. The Biological Basis of Modern Surgical Practice. 14th ed. Philadelphia: Saunders, 1991:599.

Fig. 16-2. Morris PJ, Malt RA, Oxford Textbook of Surgery. Oxford: Oxford University Press, 1994:733.

Fig. 16-3. Morris PJ, Malt RA, Oxford Textbook of Surgery. Oxford: Oxford University Press, 1994:734.

Fig. 16-4. Sabiston DC. Textbook of Surgery. The Biological Basis of Modern Surgical Practice. 14th ed. Philadelphia: Saunders, 1991:613.

Fig. 18-1. Sabiston DC. Textbook of Surgery. The Biological Basis of Modern Surgical Practice. 14th ed. Philadelphia: Saunders, 1991.

Fig. 18-2. Sabiston DC. Textbook of Surgery. The Biological Basis of Modern Surgical Practice. 14th ed. Philadelphia: Saunders, 1991.

Fig. 18-3. Way LW. Current Surgical Diagnosis and Treatment. 9th ed. Norwalk, CT: Appleton & Lange, 1991:615.

Fig. 18-4. Sabiston DC. Textbook of Surgery. The Biological Basis of Modern Surgical Practice. 14th ed. Philadelphia: Saunders, 1991.

Fig. 18-5. Sabiston DC. Textbook of Surgery. The Biological Basis of Modern Surgical Practice. 14th ed. Philadelphia: Saunders, 1991.

Fig. 18-6. Way LW. Current Surgical Diagnosis and Treatment. 9th ed. Norwalk, CT: Appleton & Lange, 1991:615.

Fig. 18-7. Sadler TW. Langman's Medical Embryology. 6th ed. Baltimore: Williams & Wilkins, 1990.

Fig. 19-1. Jarrell B. Surgery: National Medical Series (NMS). New York: Wiley, 1986:104.

Fig. 19-2. Way LW. Current Surgical Diagnosis and Treatment. 9th ed. Norwalk, CT: Appleton & Lange, 1991:461.

Fig. 19-3. Jarrell B. Surgery: National Medical Series (NMS). New York: Wiley, 1986:105.

Fig. 19-4. Morris PJ, Malt RA, Oxford Textbook of Surgery. New York: Oxford University Press, 1994:104.

Fig. 19-5. Sabiston DC. Textbook of Surgery. The Biological Basis of Modern Surgical Practice. 14th ed. Philadelphia: Saunders, 1991.

Fig. 19-6. Lawrence PF. Essentials of General Surgery. Baltimore: Williams & Wilkins, 1988:180.

Fig. 19-7. Lawrence PF. Essentials of General Surgery. Baltimore: Williams & Wilkins, 1988:181.

Fig. 19-8. Way LW. Current Surgical Diagnosis and Treatment. 9th ed. Norwalk, CT: Appleton & Lange, 1991:488.

Fig. 19-9. Morris PJ, Malt RA, Oxford Textbook of Surgery. New York: Oxford University Press, 1994:939.

Fig. 19-10. Cameron JL. Current Surgical Therapy. 5th ed. St. Louis: Mosby, 1995:92.

Fig. 19-11. Cameron JL. Current Surgical Therapy. 5th ed. St. Louis: Mosby, 1995:92.

Fig. 20-1. Way LW. Current Surgical Diagnosis and Treatment. 9th ed. Norwalk, CT: Appleton & Lange, 1991:586.

Fig. 20-2. Sabiston DC. Textbook of Surgery. The biological basis of modern surgical practice. 14th ed. Philadelphia: Saunders, 1991:1109.

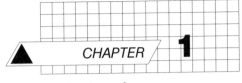

CHAPTER 1

Arteries

► ANEURYSMS AND DISSECTIONS

An aneurysm is an abnormal dilation of an artery. Saccular aneurysms occur when a portion of the artery forms an outpouching or "mushroom." Fusiform aneurysms occur when the entire arterial diameter grows. True aneurysms involve all layers of the arterial wall, intima, media, and adventitia. False aneurysms involve only the adventitia. In contrast, a dissection occurs when a defect in the intima allows blood to enter between layers of the wall (Fig. 1-1). Blood pressure then causes the layers of the wall to separate from one another. The serious nature of arterial aneurysms relates to the weakened vessel wall and potential for rupture or vascular compromise; dissections can progress to compromise the ostia of visceral arteries or can progress into the heart and compromise the coronary circulation or lead to tamponade.

Abdominal Aortic Aneurysm

Anatomy

The abdominal aorta lies below the diaphragm and above the iliac arteries. Branches include the celiac trunk, superior mesenteric artery, inferior mesenteric artery, renal arteries, and gonadal arteries. Most aneurysms begin distal to the takeoff of the renal arteries.

Etiology

Ninety-five percent of aneurysms of the abdominal aorta are due to atherosclerosis, but they can be caused by trauma, infection, syphilis, and Marfan's syndrome.

Epidemiology

Abdominal aortic aneurysms are responsible for 15,000 deaths per year; the incidence is approximately 50 per 100,000. Men are affected 10 times more frequently than women, with an age of onset usually between 50 and 70. Risk factors include atherosclerosis, hypertension, hypercholesterolemia, smoking, and obesity. The disease is associated with peripheral vascular disease, heart disease, and carotid artery disease.

History

Most aneurysms are asymptomatic. Should a catastrophic event occur, such as enlargement, rupture, or compromise of vascular supply, patients may complain of abdominal, back, chest, or flank pain. The pain usually occurs suddenly and does not remit.

Physical Examination

Abdominal examination may reveal a pulsatile abdominal mass. Factors that suggest progression, rupture, or compromise of vascular supply include tenderness, hypotension, or tachycardia. In addition, the lower extremities may have pallor, cool temperature, or pulses that are diminished or unequal.

Diagnostic Evaluation

Ultrasound is an accurate, noninvasive way to assess the size of the aneurysm and the presence of clot within the arterial lumen. Computed tomography (CT) or magnetic resonance imaging (MRI) provides anatomic detail and precise localization of the aneurysm. An aortogram is helpful in planning surgical intervention to demonstrate involvement of other vessels, specifically the renal, mesenteric, and iliac arteries.

Treatment

If the patient is asymptomatic, workup can proceed electively. Any patient presenting with symptoms or physical examination suggesting a catastrophic aortic event should undergo emergent diagnostic workup or intervention. Treatment of asymptomatic abdominal aortic aneurysms depends on the size of the lesion. The size of an aneurysm is directly proportional to its propensity to grow, leak, or rupture. Aneurysms smaller than 4 cm are unlikely to rupture, and medical management with antihypertensives, preferably beta blockers, is advocated. When the aneurysm reaches approximately 4–5 cm, operative intervention is considered with the understanding that the morbidity of the operation is significant and the mortality is approximately 1%. When the aneurysm reaches 5 cm, the incidence of rupture is greater than 25% at 5 years.

Once the diagnosis of ruptured or leaking abdominal aortic aneurysm is made, arrangements are made for fluid resuscitation and immediate operative intervention.

▲ 1

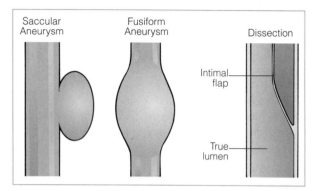

Figure 1-1 Aneurysms and dissections.

Thoracic Aortic Aneurysm

Anatomy
The thoracic aorta lies between the heart and the diaphragm. It gives rise to the subclavian arteries, carotid arteries, bronchial arteries, esophageal arteries, and intercostal arteries.

Etiology
Thoracic aortic aneurysms are caused by cystic medial necrosis, atherosclerosis and less commonly by trauma, dissection, or infection.

Epidemiology
Males are affected three times as often as females. Risk factors include atherosclerosis, smoking, hypertension, and family history.

History
Most aneurysms are asymptomatic. Rupture usually presents with chest pain or pressure. Expansion of the aneurysm can compress the trachea, leading to cough, or erode into the trachea or bronchus, causing massive hemoptysis. An aneurysm close to the aortic valve can cause dilation of the annulus, leading to aortic valve insufficiency and chest pain, dyspnea, or syncope.

Physical Examination
Hypotension and tachycardia may be present. If the aneurysm involves the aortic annulus and blood escapes into the pericardium, tamponade will ensue, characterized by Beck's triad of shock, distant heart sounds, and distended neck veins.

Diagnostic Evaluation
Chest radiography may show a widened thoracic aorta. Electrocardiogram may demonstrate myocardial ischemia, especially if the aneurysm compromises the coronary supply.

In the asymptomatic patient with a thoracic aneurysm, CT or echocardiography is helpful in establishing the diagnosis. Echocardiography can also determine the extent of involvement of the aortic valve and possible cardiac tamponade. Aortography is necessary for planning operative intervention because it defines the relation of a number of critical structures to the aneurysm.

Treatment
As with abdominal aortic aneurysms, operative repair should be considered when the maximum diameter approaches 5 cm. Symptomatic presentation is an indication for immediate operative intervention.

Aortic Dissection

Pathogenesis
Dissections are often due to trauma but can be caused by hypertension, Marfan's syndrome, or aortic coarctation.

Epidemiology
These are more common than either thoracic or abdominal aneurysms. Incidence increases with age, and males are more commonly affected than females.

History
Patients usually complain of the immediate onset of horrible pain, usually in the chest, back, or abdomen. Nausea or lightheadedness may also be present.

Physical Examination
Patients may be hypotensive. Rales on chest auscultation or a new aortic murmur suggest the dissection continued retrograde into the aortic root. Peripheral pulses will be diminished if distal blood flow is compromised. If the dissection continued into the visceral arteries, compromise of mesenteric vessels can produce abdominal pain, compromise of renal arteries can cause oliguria, and compromise of spinal blood supply can produce neurologic deficits.

Diagnostic Evaluation
A chest radiograph may show a widened mediastinum. CT may show the dissection or clot in the arterial lumen. Diagnosis can be made with transesophageal ultrasound, MRI, or aortogram.

Treatment
Dissection of the ascending thoracic aorta requires surgery because of the potential for retrograde progression into the aortic root and subsequent compromise of the coronary circulation or tamponade from rupture into the pericardium. Antihypertensive therapy is used

preoperatively in an attempt to halt the progression of the dissection. Abdominal aortic dissections can be managed with antihypertensives, including sodium nitroprusside and beta blockade. Invasive monitoring with fluid resuscitation should be instituted immediately, with surgery dependent on further progression of the lesion.

Key Points

1. Aneurysms and dissections can be rapidly fatal.
2. Operative repair should be considered for asymptomatic aneurysms greater than 4 or 5 cm.
3. Symptomatic aneurysms or dissections require emergent diagnosis and treatment.

▶ CAROTID ARTERY DISEASE

Anatomy

The common carotid artery on the right arises from the brachiocephalic artery and on the left from the left subclavian artery. The common carotid then bifurcates into internal and external branches. The internal carotid gives off the ophthalmic artery before continuing to the circle of Willis to supply the brain.

Pathogenesis

Symptoms are the result of atherosclerosis. Mechanisms of morbidity include plaque rupture, ulceration, hemorrhage, thrombosis, and low flow states. Because of the rich collateralization of the cerebral circulation through the circle of Willis, thrombosis and low flow states may be asymptomatic.

Epidemiology

Atherosclerotic occlusive disease of the carotid artery is an important cause of stroke. Four hundred thousand people are hospitalized annually for stroke, and cerebrovascular events are the third most common cause of death in the United States. The incidence of stroke increases with age. Other risk factors include hypertension, diabetes, smoking, and hypercholesterolemia. Markers for carotid disease include evidence of other atherosclerotic disease and prior neurologic events.

History

Patients will often relate previous neurologic events, including focal motor deficits, weakness, clumsiness, and expressive or cognitive aphasia. These may occur as a transient ischemic attack (TIA), which resolves in 24 hours, a reversible ischemic neurologic deficit, which resolves in greater than 24 hours, or a fixed neurologic deficit. A characteristic presentation for ca-

rotid disease is amaurosis fugax, or transient monocular blindness, usually described as a "shade" being pulled down in front of the patient's eye. This is due to occlusion of a branch of the ophthalmic artery.

Physical Examination

Patients may exhibit a fixed neurologic deficit. Hollenhorst plaques on retinal examination are evidence of previous emboli. A carotid bruit is evidence of turbulence in carotid blood flow, but the presence of a bruit does not unequivocally translate into a hemodynamically significant lesion and the absence of a bruit does not unequivocally indicate the absence of significant disease.

Diagnostic Evaluation

Carotid duplex scanning is both sensitive and specific for carotid disease. Conventional or magnetic resonance angiogram is more accurate for assessing the degree of stenosis.

Treatment

Treatment depends on the history, degree of stenosis, and characteristics of the plaque. Antiplatelet therapy with aspirin is effective in preventing neurologic events. When dealing with an acute event, heparin should be considered after head CT determines that the event is not hemorrhagic.

Indications for carotid endarterectomy are controversial. Patients offered operation include those with greater than 75% stenosis, 70% stenosis and symptoms, bilateral disease and symptoms, and greater than 50% stenosis and recurring TIAs despite aspirin therapy.

Key Point

Carotid artery disease

1. Is a major cause of morbidity and mortality in the United States.

▶ ACUTE AND CHRONIC MESENTERIC VASCULAR DISEASE

Anatomy

This category includes disease of the celiac axis, which supplies the liver, spleen, pancreas, and stomach; the superior mesenteric artery, which supplies the pancreas, small bowel, and proximal colon; and inferior mesenteric artery, which supplies the distal colon and rectum.

Pathogenesis

Acute ischemia may be associated with embolic events secondary to atherosclerotic disease or mural cardiac thrombus. In addition, vasopressor agents can produce acute ischemia.

Chronic ischemia usually requires severe atherosclerotic disease in at least two major arterial trunks among the superior and inferior mesenteric arteries and the celiac axis because of the extensive collateralization.

Epidemiology

The incidence of acute ischemia is estimated at 1 of 1,000 hospital admissions and mortality is over 50%. Chronic ischemia increases with age, and risk factors include hypertension, smoking, hypercholesterolemia, and diabetes.

History

Patients with **acute ischemia** may describe previous embolic events, atrial fibrillation, or congestive failure. Abdominal pain is usually sudden in onset and severe with diarrhea or vomiting.

History in **chronic mesenteric ischemia** usually reveals crampy abdominal pain after eating. This results in decreased oral intake and weight loss. Nausea, vomiting, constipation, or diarrhea may occur. The disease can be mistaken for malignant disease or cholelithiasis.

Physical Examination

In episodes of **acute ischemia,** the classic finding is "pain out of proportion to physical examination." The abdomen may be distended. Rectal examination often reveals guaiac positive stool. Atrial fibrillation may be present. Physical findings in **chronic ischemia** include abdominal bruits, guaiac positive stool, and evidence of peripheral vascular disease or coronary artery disease.

Diagnostic Evaluation

In **acute ischemia** there may be an elevated white blood cell count, metabolic acidosis, or an elevated hematocrit as fluid is sequestered in the infarcting bowel. Abdominal radiographs are often normal in the early phase of the disease, but as the intestine becomes edematous, "thumbprinting" of the bowel wall occurs. Evaluation in **chronic ischemia** includes selective visceral angiography to identify the site of the lesion.

Treatment

Once the diagnosis of **acute ischemia** is made, laparotomy with examination and resection of any infarcted bowel should proceed urgently. Despite aggressive intervention, mortality is extremely high. For chronic ischemia, angiogram will define the lesion and allow consideration of surgical options.

Key Points

1. Acute mesenteric ischemia presents with "pain out of proportion to examination" and a mechanism for embolic disease is usually present.
2. Chronic mesenteric ischemia results in weight loss and abdominal pain and is frequently mistaken for malignant disease.

▶ PERIPHERAL VASCULAR DISEASE

Anatomy

Lesions may occur in the iliac, common and superficial femoral, popliteal, peroneal, anterior tibial, and posterior tibial arteries.

Pathogenesis

For **acute disease,** an embolus causes a sudden decrease in blood flow. The most common sources are the aorta and heart.

For **chronic disease,** progressive atherosclerotic disease causes narrowing of the arterial lumen and decreased blood flow. Pain occurs as decreased blood flow is unable to meet the metabolic and waste removal demand of the tissue.

Epidemiology

Acute disease occurs in patients with cardiac thrombus, atrial fibrillation, or atherosclerosis.

Risk factors for **chronic disease** include evidence of atherosclerosis, smoking, diabetes, hypertension, and advanced age.

History

Acute ischemia causes sudden and severe lower extremity pain and paresthesia.

Chronic ischemia typically presents with claudication, defined as reproducible pain on exercise relieved by rest. The site of claudication provides a clue to the level of disease. Buttock claudication usually indicates aortoiliac disease, whereas calf claudication suggests femoral atherosclerosis. Pain at rest is indicative of severe disease and a threatened limb. There may be slow or nonhealing ulcers. Patients will commonly have other atherosclerotic disease.

Physical Examination

In **acute disease,** the patient may exhibit pulselessness, pallor, and poikilothermia (coolness). Taken together with pain and paresthesia, these form the 5 p's of acute vascular compromise (Fig. 1-2). For

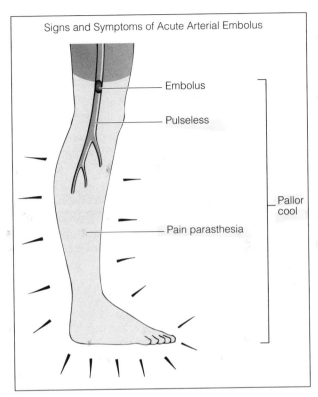

Signs and Symptoms of Acute Arterial Embolus

- Embolus
- Pulseless
- Pallor cool
- Pain parasthesia

Figure 1-2 Signs and symptoms of acute arterial embolus.

chronic disease, the lower extremity may reveal loss of hair, pallor on elevation, rubor on placing the extremity in a dependent position, wasting of musculature, thick nails, and thin skin. The extremity may be cool to the touch, and pulses may be diminished or absent. Ulcers or frank necrosis may be present.

Diagnostic Evaluation

Angiogram is necessary in cases of acute ischemia to identify the lesion.

Evaluation for chronic ischemia include Doppler flow measurement of distal pulses. The normal signal is triphasic; as disease progresses, the signal becomes biphasic, monophasic, and then absent. Ankle-brachial indices of less than 0.5 are indicative of significant disease. Arteriography is the gold standard for defining the level and extent of disease and for planning surgery.

Treatment

Acute ischemic embolus can be treated with heparin, thrombolysis, or embolectomy. For patients with chronic ischemia, those with claudication have a low rate of limb loss, and initial therapy is based on smoking cessation and a graded exercise program. Success rates with nonoperative therapy is good. In patients with disabling claudication, threatened limbs, non-healing ulcers or gangrene, angioplasty or revascularization should be considered (Fig. 1-3).

Key Points

1. Acute peripheral embolus is marked by the 5 p's.

2. Symptoms of chronic peripheral vascular disease usually follow a well-defined progression.

3. Operation should be considered only in patients with severe chronic peripheral vascular disease.

Figure 1-3 Progression of peripheral vascular disease.

	Claudication	Rest Pain	Gangrene
Blood Flow	Decreased	Markedly decreased	Minimal
ABI	About 0.5	0.3 to 0.5	Less than 0.3
Treatment	Smoking cessation Graded exercise	? Revascularization ? Angioplasty	Amputation ? Revascularization ? Angioplasty

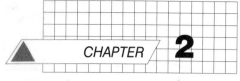
Breast

Thoracodorsal n — latissimus dorsi — Shoulder AB
Long Thoracic n — serratus ant. — winged scapula

► ANATOMY AND PHYSIOLOGY

The breast is composed of glandular tissue dorsal to the pectoralis major muscle. Support is provided by Cooper's ligaments. The functional units are lobules that contain terminal ducts where milk is produced and ductules and ducts that convey the milk to the nipple. The lymphatic drainage travels through axillary, mammary, and central nodes along the axillary vein and medially to the internal mammary nodes. Nodes are characterized based on their relation to the pectoralis minor. Level 1 nodes are lateral to the muscle, level 2 nodes are beneath it, and level 3 nodes are medial to it. In the axilla lie the thoracodorsal nerve, which provides motor function to the latissimus dorsi; and the long thoracic nerve, which provides motor function to the serratus anterior. Damage to these nerves during dissection leads to weakness in shoulder abduction and a winged scapula, respectively.

► PATHOLOGY

Benign breast lesions include simple cysts, fibroadenomas, "fibrocystic disease," and papillomas. Fibrocystic disease comprises a group of findings that include firm nodular lesions, cyst formation, and epithelial hyperplasia. Tumors with low malignant potential include Phylloides tumors. The most common malignant lesions are lobular and ductal carcinoma. These occur in noninvasive or in situ form that do not penetrate the basement membrane and invasive forms that do. Inflammatory breast cancer is characterized by tumor invasion of lymphatic channels. Paget's disease occurs when tumor cells invade the epidermal layer of the skin.

► EPIDEMIOLOGY

Breast cancer is the second leading cause of cancer deaths among women. It is estimated that between 1 in 9 and 1 in 11 women will be diagnosed with breast cancer during their lifetime. Significant risk factors include age (breast cancer before age 30 is rare), history of breast cancer in a first-degree relative (two to three times normal risk, higher if the relative had premenopausal cancer), and atypical hyperplasia diagnosed on previous biopsy (four times normal risk). In addition, personal history of breast cancer and lobular carcinoma in situ are risk factors for invasive cancer. Less important risk factors include early menarche and late menopause. Ductal carcinoma is the most common breast malignancy. Simple cysts, fibroadenomas, fibrocystic change, and papillomas are not associated with increased risk of breast cancer. Fibroadenoma is the most common tumor of young women. Intraductal papilloma is the most common cause of bloody nipple discharge.

► HISTORY

Women with breast cancer may relate the discovery of a new mass. Malignant lesions are usually not cyclic with menses, whereas simple cysts are. Masses that increase in size are more concerning. Constitutional symptoms may include weight loss, nausea, and malaise. Bone pain is an ominous symptom that may signify skeletal metastases. Intraductal papilloma may present with nipple discharge. Patients with inflammatory cancer may describe warmth or tenderness at the site.

► PHYSICAL EXAMINATION

Breast asymmetry, dimpling or retractions, and excoriation or edema of the skin are extremely sensitive for malignancy. Fibroadenomas are usually well circumscribed and mobile. Characteristics of malignancy on palpation include firmness and indistinct borders. Lymphadenopathy may be present, and there may be bloody discharge. Inflammatory cancer may display erythema and skin excoriation, termed peau d'orange. Paget's disease may present with nipple or areolar excoriation. Phylloides tumors usually present with a painless mass.

► DIAGNOSTIC EVALUATION

Screening mammography has been shown by a number of studies to decrease mortality from breast cancer, however, a normal mammogram in the setting of a palpable mass does not exclude a cancer. The current recommendations from the American Cancer Society are for a baseline mammogram between the ages of 35 and 39 and then every 1–2 years between the ages of 40 and 50 and yearly after age 50. Characteristics on mammogram that are suspicious for malignancy include densities with irregular margins, spiculated lesions, microcalcifications, or rod-like or branching patterns. Any changes from a previous mammogram should be viewed with concern, and any suspicious mass should be considered for biopsy. Needle-directed biopsy is useful for nonpalpable mammographic abnormalities. This technique uses mammographic guidance to place a needle at the lesion that the surgeon uses to locate it. Palpable masses should be considered for fine-needle aspiration. Cancer is unlikely if all of the following criteria are met: the mass completely disappears after aspiration, does not return, and if the fluid is Hemoccult negative. If any of these criteria are not met, open excisional biopsy should be performed. Aspirate should be sent for cytology, which has a sensitivity of 70–90% depending on the cytologist and the surgeon.

▶ TREATMENT

For ductal carcinoma in situ, total mastectomy carries almost 100% cure rate. Breast conserving therapy (lumpectomy) with radiation therapy and careful follow-up is usually also offered. Patients with LCIS are usually given careful follow-up care, but bilateral prophylactic mastectomies may be offered in some circumstances. These include preference for a definitive procedure to the uncertainty of follow-up care, inability to follow-up, or a strong family history of breast cancer.

Treatment options for stage I or II cancer include modified radical mastectomy or lumpectomy with axillary node dissection and breast irradiation. Modified radical mastectomy involves removal of all breast tissue and axillary node dissection, sparing all motor nerves and muscles of the chest wall. Lumpectomy involves resection of the mass. Patients with lumpectomy alone have equal survival but higher local recurrence rates, but adding radiation therapy to lumpectomy decreases the recurrence rate to equal mastectomy. Axillary node dissection allows staging and guides treatment. Chemotherapy and radiation are offered according to Table 2-3.

For patients with stage III or IV disease, surgical resection for local control and radiation or chemotherapy have all been shown to be of benefit (see Table 2-3). Because surgery treats only the local manifestations of a disseminated disease, resection should not be the basis of treatment.

Phylloides tumors and sarcomas are treated with wide excision.

TABLE 2-1
TNM Staging for Breast Cancer

Stage	Description
Tumor	
TX	Primary tumor not assessable
TO	No evidence of primary tumor
Tis	Carcinoma in situ
T1	Tumor 2 cm or less in greatest dimension
T2	Tumor more than 2 cm but not more than 5 cm in greatest dimension
T3	Tumor more than 5 cm in greatest dimension
T4	Tumor of any size with direct extension into chest wall (not including pectoral muscles) or skin edema or skin ulceration or satellite skin nodules confined to the same breast or inflammatory carcinoma
Regional lymph nodes	
NX	Regional lymph nodes not assessable
NO	No regional lymph node involvement
N1	Metastasis to movable ipsilateral axillary lymph node(s)
N2	Metastasis to ipsilateral axillary lymph node(s) fixed to one another or to other structures
N3	Metastasis to ipsilateral internal mammary lymph nodes
Distant metastasis	
MX	Presence of distant metastasis cannot be assessed
MO	No distant metastasis
M1	Distant metastasis present (including ipsilateral supraclavicular lymph nodes)

TABLE 2-2
AJCC Classification for Breast Cancer Based on TNM Criteria

Stage	Tumor	Nodes	Metastases
O	Tis	NO	MO
I	T1	NO	MO
IIA	TO, 1	N1	MO
	T2	NO	MO
IIB	T2	N1	MO
	T3	NO	MO
IIIA	TO, 1, 2	N2	MO
	T3	N1, 2	MO
IIIB	T4	N1, 2	MO
	Any T	N3	MO
IV	Any T	Any N	M1

TABLE 2-3

Current Recommendations for Adjuvant Therapy in Stage I and II Breast Cancer

Tumor	Premenopausal Patient		Postmenopausal Patient	
	ER Positive	ER Negative	ER Positive	ER Negative
<1 cm, negative nodes	NT	NT	NT	NT
≥1 cm, negative nodes	TAM ± chemo	CHEMO	TAM ± chemo	CHEMO
Positive nodes	CHEMO*	CHEMO*	TAM ± chemo	CHEMO*

NT, no treatment indicated outside of a clinical study; TAM, treatment with tamoxifen for at least 5 years indicated; chemo, chemo may be indicated for some patients in addition to or instead of tamoxifen; CHEMO, chemotherapy is indicated.
*Adjuvant treatment has been proved to improve overall survival.

▶ PROGNOSIS

Patients with stage I disease have an approximately 80% 5-year disease-free survival, stage II disease carries a 60% 5-year disease-free survival, whereas stage III disease portends only a 20% 5-year disease-free survival. Patients with stage IV disease have minimal long-term survival. The presence of estrogen and progesterone receptors independently carry improved survival.

▶ KEY POINTS

1. Breast cancer is the second leading cause of cancer deaths among women.

2. Significant risk factors include age, family or personal history, atypical hyperplasia on biopsy, and lobular carcinoma in situ.

3. Mammography decreases mortality. Current recommendations are for a baseline study between 35 and 39 years of age and then every 1–2 years between the ages of 40 and 50, and every year thereafter.

4. A palpable abnormality should not be dismissed because of a normal mammogram, and a mammographic abnormality should not be dismissed because the mass is not palpable.

5. Treatment options for DCIS include mastectomy or lumpectomy and radiation.

6. Axillary node dissection is useful in patients with invasive cancer for staging which will guide treatment.

7. Surgical options for invasive cancer include modified radical mastectomy or lumpectomy with axillary node dissection and radiation.

Handwritten notes:

ImV → splenic V.;
↳SmV → Portal v.;
LIVER

Anastomosis q Rislan → SmA ; IMA

Ileocolic → ® colic → middle colic → Sup. Mesenteric
(cecum
Ascending
Mid-transverse)

① colic → Sigmoid → sup. hemorrhoidal → Inf. mesenteric
Iliac → middle
Inferior hemorrhoidal → (Rectal)
(mid-transv.
Sigmoid
Rectum)

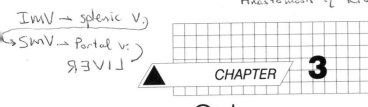

CHAPTER 3

Colon

▶ ANATOMY AND PHYSIOLOGY

The colon begins at the ileocecal valve and extends to the anal canal. Its primary function is the reabsorption of water and sodium, secretion of potassium and bicarbonate, and storage of fecal material. The ascending and descending colon are fixed in a retroperitoneal location, whereas the remainder of the colon is intraperitoneal. Arterial supply to the cecum, ascending colon, and the midtransverse colon is from the superior mesenteric artery (SMA) by way of the ileocolic, right colic, and middle colic arteries. The remainder of the colon is supplied by the inferior mesenteric artery (IMA) by way of the left colic, sigmoid, and superior hemorrhoidal arteries. The middle and inferior hemorrhoidal arteries contribute to rectal blood flow, arising from the iliac circulation. The long anastomosis between the SMA and IMA is called the anastomosis of Riolan, and the arcades in proximity to the mesenteric border of the colon are referred to as the marginal artery of Drummond (Fig. 3-1). Venous drainage from the colon includes the superior and inferior mesenteric veins. The IMV joins the splenic vein and then the SMV to form the portal vein, which enters the liver. In this way, the liver is allowed first pass to detoxify and sterilize blood before it enters the central circulation. Lymphatic drainage follows the arteries and veins.

▶ ULCERATIVE COLITIS

Ulcerative colitis is an inflammatory disease of the colon with unknown etiology. It almost always involves the rectum and extends backward toward the cecum to varying degrees.

Pathology

Inflammation is confined to the mucosa and submucosa. Superficial ulcers, thickened mucosa, crypt abscesses and pseudopolyps may also be present.

Epidemiology

The incidence is 6 per 100,000. The disease commonly presents in the third or fourth decade. It is more common in developed countries, whites, and Jews. There is no predilection for sex. Approximately 20% of patients will have first-degree relatives who are affected. Linkage analysis has identified an association with HLA AW24 and BW25.

History

Patients commonly complain of bloody diarrhea, fever, abdominal pain, and weight loss. Multiple attacks are common. A number of diseases are associated with ulcerative colitis, including sclerosing cholangitis in 1% of patients, arthritis, iritis, cholangitis, aphthous ulcers, and ankylosing spondylosis, and these diseases may be part of the initial presentation.

Physical Examination

Abdominal pain is common. Rectal tenderness may occur with rectal fissures. The disease may present with abdominal distention as evidence of massive colonic distention, a situation known as toxic megacolon. This may progress to frank perforation with signs of peritonitis.

Diagnostic Evaluation

Colonoscopy may demonstrate thickened, friable mucosa. Fissures and pseudopolyps, if present, almost always involve the rectum and varying portions of the colon. Biopsy shows ulceration limited to the mucosa and submucosa; crypt abscesses may be present. Barium enema may reveal a stovepipe colon with smooth edges and ulcers.

Complications

Patients may develop perforation or obstruction from stricture. Hemorrhage or toxic megacolon are uncommon. Colon cancer occurs frequently, with a risk of approximately 10% within 20 years.

Treatment

Initial therapy is medical, with fluid administration, electrolyte correction, and parenteral nutrition if necessary. Steroids, other immunosuppressives, and sulfasalazine are all effective. Indications for surgery include colonic obstruction, massive blood loss, failure of medical therapy, toxic megacolon, and cancer. The recommendation of prophylactic colectomy for these patients is being reconsidered based on recent data suggesting the incidence of cancer is not as high as once thought. With sphincter sparing operations, continence and bowel movements can be preserved.

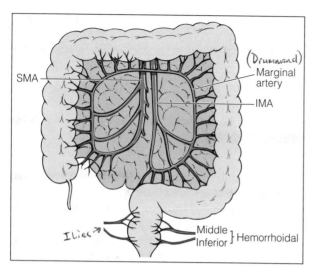

Figure 3-1 Arterial supply of the colon.

Key Points

1. Ulcerative colitis presents with bloody diarrhea and abdominal pain. Pathologic changes are limited to the mucosa and submucosa.

2. Patients with ulcerative colitis have a significant risk of colon cancer.

3. Surgery for ulcerative colitis is used for intractable bleeding, obstruction, failure of medical therapy, toxic megacolon, and risk of cancer.

▶ DIVERTICULOSIS

Diverticula are outpouchings of the colon. They occur at points where the arterial supply penetrates the bowel wall. Most are false diverticula because all layers of the bowel wall are not included. Diverticulosis refers to the presence of diverticula. Most diverticula are in the sigmoid colon. Diverticulosis is the most common cause of lower gastrointestinal hemorrhage, most commonly from the right colon. Only 15% of people with diverticula will ever have a significant episode of bleeding.

Epidemiology

Diverticular disease is common in developed nations and is likely related to low fiber diets. Men and women are equally affected, and the prevalence increases dramatically with age. Approximately one third of the population has diverticular disease, but this number increases to over one half of those over 80.

History

Patients usually present with bleeding per rectum without other complaints. There may have been previous episodes of bleeding or crampy abdominal pain, commonly in the left lower quadrant.

Diagnostic Evaluation

For patients who stop bleeding spontaneously, elective colonoscopy should be performed to determine the etiology of the bleeding. If bleeding continues, diagnostic and therapeutic modalities include radioisotope bleeding scans, which have variable success rates, and mesenteric angiography, which has excellent success rates in the presence of active bleeding.

Treatment

Asymptomatic individuals require no treatment. Eighty percent of bleeding will stop spontaneously. Elective segmental or subtotal colectomy may be offered after a first episode, depending on the ability to accurately determine the site of bleeding, the severity of the initial presentation, and the general status of the patient. Patients with recurrent bleeding are usually offered surgical resection. Active bleeding is treated colonoscopically if the colon can be cleaned. Embolization of the bleeding vessel may be possible using angiography. If these methods fail and no bleeding site is identified, emergent subtotal colectomy is performed, which involves removal of the entire colon. If the bleeding site is identified, segmental colectomy can be performed, usually based on the arterial branch feeding the bleeding site.

Key Points

1. Diverticulosis is the most common cause of lower gastrointestinal bleeding.

2. Surgical therapy for diverticulosis is recommended for recurrent or intractable bleeding.

▶ DIVERTICULITIS

The narrow neck of the diverticula predisposes to infection, which occurs either from increased intraluminal pressure or inspissated food particles. Infection leads to localized or free perforation into the abdomen. Diverticulitis most commonly occurs in the sigmoid and is rare in the right colon. Approximately 20% of patients with diverticula will experience an episode of diverticulitis. Each attack makes a subsequent attack more likely and increases the risk of complications.

History

Patients usually present with left lower quadrant pain; less commonly right-sided diverticulitis causes right-sided pain. The pain usually is progressive over a few days and may be associated with diarrhea or constipation.

Physical Examination

Abdominal tenderness, most commonly in the left lower quadrant, is the most common finding. There may be local peritoneal signs of rebound and guarding. Diffuse rebound tenderness or guarding as evidence of diffuse peritonitis suggests free intra-abdominal perforation.

Diagnostic Evaluation

The white blood cell count is usually elevated. Radiographs of the abdomen are usually normal. Computed tomography (CT) may demonstrate pericolic fat stranding, bowel wall thickening, and an abscess. Colonoscopy and barium enema should not be performed during an acute episode because of the risk of causing or exacerbating an existing perforation.

Complications

Patients may develop stricture, perforation, or fistulization with the bladder, skin, vagina, or other portions of the bowel.

Treatment

Most episodes of diverticulitis are mild and can be treated on an outpatient basis with broad-spectrum oral antibiotics. Ciprofloxacin and flagyl would be an appropriate choice to cover bowel flora. For severe cases or cases in elderly or debilitated patients, hospitalization with bowel rest and broad-spectrum intravenous antibiotics (e.g., ampicillin, gentamycin, and flagyl) are required. For patients who do not improve in 48 hours on this regimen, CT-guided abscess drainage may obviate the need for emergent operation. In the event of free perforation or failure of the modalities discussed, surgical drainage with colostomy is required. In addition, surgical resection is indicated in the presence of the complications described above and after a second attack because the risk of subsequent attacks increases; the risk of complications with a second attack is 60%.

Key Points

1. Diverticulitis usually presents with left lower quadrant pain.
2. Surgical therapy for diverticulitis is indicated after a second attack because of the high recurrence and complication rate.

▶ COLONIC NEOPLASMS

Recent evidence suggests colon cancer follows an orderly progression in which adenomatous polyps undergo malignant transformation over a variable time period. For this reason, polyps are considered premalignant lesions. Fifty percent of carcinomas will have a ras gene mutation, whereas 75% will have a p53 gene mutation.

Epidemiology

Colon cancer is the second most common cause of cancer death in the United States. Risk factors include high fat and low fiber diets, age, and family history. Ulcerative colitis, Crohn disease, and Gardner's syndrome all predispose to cancer, and all patients with familial polyposis coli will develop cancer if not treated.

Pathology

Polyps are tubular or villous, with some lesions exhibiting features of both. Villous adenomas more commonly harbor malignant regions. As each grows in size, the likelihood of it having undergone malignant transformation increases significantly. Although tubular adenomas under 1 cm contain malignancy in only 1% of cases, lesions greater than 2 cm contain malignancy 35% of the time. For villous adenomas, the numbers are 10 and 50%. Ninety percent of colon cancers are adenocarcinomas and 20% of these are mucinous, which carry worse prognosis. Other types include squamous, adenosquamous, lymphoma, sarcoma, and carcinoid.

Screening

Screening is aimed at detecting polyps and early malignant lesions. The current screening recommendations from the American Cancer Society for patients who are asymptomatic and without risk factors include digital rectal examination every year beginning at 40 and fecal occult blood test every year beginning at 50 with sigmoidoscopy every 3–5 years beginning at 50. For patients with first-degree relatives diagnosed with colon cancer before age 55, colonoscopy every 5 years is also recommended.

Staging

Staging of colon cancer follows Dukes staging (Table 3-1). Dukes A lesions are limited to the mucosa without lymph node involvement. Dukes B1 lesions involve the muscularis; whereas B2 lesions involve the serosa and B3 lesions extend to adjacent organs. B lesions have no lymph node involvement. Dukes C1 lesions involve mucosa or muscularis, whereas C2 lesions involve the serosa; both include lymph nodes with disease. Dukes D lesions are metastatic. Approximate survival rates at 5 years for A lesions are 95%, for B1 lesions 85%, for B2 lesions 65%, for C1 lesions 55%, and

> **TABLE 3-1**
>
> ## TNM Staging Classification of Colorectal Cancer*

Stage	Description
TNM system	
Primary tumor (T)	
TX	Primary tumor cannot be assessed
TO	No evidence of tumor in resected specimen (prior polypectomy or fulguration)
Tis	Carcinoma in situ
T1	Invades into submucosa
T2	Invades into muscularis propria
T3/T4	Depends on whether serosa is present
Serosa present	
T3	Invades through muscularis propria into subserosa Invades serosa (but not through) Invades pericolic fat within the leaves of the mesentery
T4	Invades through serosa into free peritoneal cavity, or through serosa into a contiguous organ
No serosa (distal two thirds of rectum, posterior left or right colon)	
T3	Invades through muscularis propria
T4	Invades other organs (vagina, prostate, ureter, kidney)
Regional lymph nodes (N)	
NX	Nodes cannot be assessed (e.g., local excision only)
NO	No regional node metastases
N1	1–3 positive nodes
N2	4 or more positive nodes
N3	Central nodes positive
Distant metastases (M)	
MX	Presence of distant metastases cannot be assessed
MO	No distant metastases
M1	Distant metastases present
Dukes staging system correlated with TNM	
Dukes A	T1, NO, MO T2, NO, MO
Dukes B	T3, NO, MO T4, NO, MO
Dukes C	T (any), N1, MO; T (any), N2, MO
Dukes D	T (any), N (any), M1
Modified Astler-Coller (MAC) system correlated with TNM	
MAC A	T1, NO, MO
MAC B1	T2, NO, MO
MAC B2	T3, NO, MO; T4, NO, MO
MAC B3	T4, NO, MO
MAC C1	T2, N1, MO; T2, N2, MO
MAC C2	T3, N1, MO; T3, N2, MO T4, N1, MO; T4, N2, MO
MAC C3	T4, N1, MO; T4, N2, MO

*In all pathologic staging systems, particularly those applied to rectal cancer, the abbreviations *m* and *g* may be used; m denotes microscopic transmural penetration; g or m + g denotes transmural penetration visible on gross inspection and confirmed microscopically.

for C2 lesions 25%. Stage D lesions have poor long-term survival.

History

Small neoplasms are often asymptomatic. Occult blood in the stool may be the only sign. As the size of the lesion grows, right colon lesions usually cause more significant bleeding, whereas lesions in the left colon typically present with obstructive symptoms, including a change in stool caliber, tenesmus, or constipation. Frank obstruction may also occur. Any lesion may produce crampy abdominal pain. Perforation causes peritonitis. Constitutional symptoms including weight loss, anorexia, and fatigue are common.

Physical Examination

Rectal examination may reveal occult or gross blood. A mass may be palpable on abdominal examination. Stigmata of hereditary disorders including familial polyposis syndrome or Gardner's syndrome may be present.

Diagnostic Evaluation

Evaluation includes a hematocrit, which may show anemia. Carcinoembryonic antigen (CEA) should be drawn, because though not a useful screening test, it is valuable as a marker for recurrent cancer. The liver is the most common site for metastases, and liver function tests can be abnormal in this case. Barium enema is an excellent test to demonstrate malignancy. Colonoscopy has the advantage of allowing biopsy or total excision of a lesion. CT is useful to evaluate for extent of disease and the presence of metastases.

Treatment

Therapy of colon cancer is based on surgical removal of the lesion. If the lesion can be removed endoscopically and pathologic evaluation reveals carcinoma in situ and complete excision, treatment is considered complete. For lesions that cannot be removed endoscopically, bowel resection is required. Segmental colon resection based on blood supply and lymphatic drainage is undertaken after suitable mechanical and antimicrobial cleansing. For lesions that lie close to the anus, anastomosis may not be possible and colostomy may be necessary. For stage C and probably stage B lesions, chemotherapy with 5-fluorouracil (5-FU) and levamisole is of benefit. Liver metastases should be resected if they number three or less and they are easily accessible.

Key Points

1. Colon cancer follows a progression from adenoma to carcinoma.
2. Adenomatous polyps are considered premalignant and must be removed entirely.
3. Screening for colon cancer involves yearly digital rectal examination beginning at age 40, yearly stool test for occult blood beginning at age 50, and sigmoidoscopy every 3–5 years beginning at age 50.

► ARTERIOVENOUS MALFORMATIONS

These lesions are being recognized with increasing frequency as a significant source of lower gastrointestinal hemorrhage. They most commonly occur in the cecum and right colon.

Epidemiology

They are one of the most common causes of lower gastrointestinal bleeding. The prevalence increases with age, so that approximately one fourth of elderly people have arteriovenous malformations.

History

Patients usually present with multiple episodes of low grade bleeding. Ten percent of the time, patients will present with massive bleeding.

Diagnostic Evaluation

Diagnosis can be made with arteriogram, nuclear scans, or colonoscopy.

Treatment

Endoscopy with laser ablation, electrocoagulation, or angiography with vasopressin is often effective. Because 80% of lesions will rebleed, definitive treatment, which may require segmental colectomy, is recommended in most cases.

Key Point

1. Arteriovenous malformations are common in the elderly and are one of the most common causes of lower gastrointestinal bleeding (LGIB).

► VOLVULUS

A volvulus occurs when a portion of colon rotates on the axis of its mesentery, compromising blood flow and creating a closed loop obstruction (Fig. 3-2).

Figure 3-2 Volvulus.

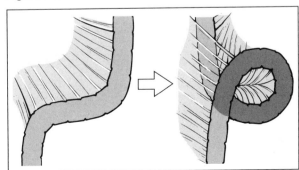

Because of their relative redundancy, the sigmoid (75%) and cecum (25%) are most commonly involved.

Epidemiology

The incidence of volvulus is approximately 2 in 100,000. Risk factors include age, chronic constipation, previous abdominal surgery, and neuropsychiatric disorders.

History

The patient usually relates the acute onset of crampy abdominal pain and distention.

Physical Examination

The abdomen is tender and distended, and peritoneal signs of rebound and involuntary guarding may be present. Frank peritonitis and shock may follow.

Diagnostic Evaluation

Abdominal radiographs may reveal a massively distended colon and a bird's beak at the point of obstruction.

Treatment

Sigmoid volvulus may be reduced by rectal tube, enemas, or proctoscopy. Because of the high rate of recurrence, operative repair after the initial resolution is recommended. Treatment of cecal volvulus is usually operative at the outset as nonoperative intervention is rarely successful.

Key Points

1. Volvulus is a life-threatening condition that presents with abdominal pain and distention.
2. KUB is diagnostic.

▶ APPENDICITIS

Appendicitis is the most common reason for urgent abdominal operation.

Epidemiology

Young adults are most commonly affected. Approximately 10% of people will develop appendicitis over their lifetime.

History

Patients typically complain of epigastric pain that migrates to the right lower quadrant. Anorexia is an almost universal complaint. The presence of generalized abdominal pain may signify rupture.

Physical Examination

Nearly all patients have right lower quadrant tenderness, classically located at McBurney's point, which is between the umbilicus and anterior superior iliac spine. Rebound and guarding develop as the disease progresses and the peritoneum becomes inflamed. Low grade fever is common. Rectal examination may reveal tenderness or a mass. Higher fever is associated with perforation. Signs of peritoneal irritation include the obturator sign, which is pain on external rotation of the flexed thigh, and the psoas sign, which is pain on right thigh flexion.

Diagnostic Evaluation

The white blood cell count is usually mildly elevated; high elevations are not usually seen unless perforation has occurred. Twenty-five percent of patients will have abnormal urinalysis. Ultrasonographic evidence of appendicitis includes wall thickening, luminal distention, and lack of compressibility. Ultrasound is also useful for demonstrating ovarian pathology, which is in the differential diagnosis of patients with right lower quadrant pain. Barium enema will often show nonfilling of the appendix. CT may show inflammation in the area of the appendix.

Treatment

Uncomplicated appendicitis requires appendectomy. Selected adults with appendiceal abscess who are clinically improving may be managed nonoperatively with antibiotics with or without CT-guided drainage. Children with perforated appendicitis require appendectomy with drainage of any abscess cavities.

Key Point

1. Appendicitis is the most common reason for urgent abdominal operation.

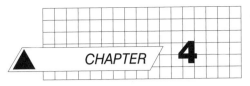

CHAPTER 4

Pituitary Gland

▶ ANATOMY AND PHYSIOLOGY

The pituitary gland is located at the base of the skull within the sella turcica, a hollow in the sphenoid bone. The optic chiasm lies anterior, the hypothalamus above, and cranial nerves III, IV, V, and VI and the carotid arteries lie in proximity. These structures are all at risk for compression or invasion from a pituitary tumor. Visual field defects can occur when a tumor encroaches on the optic chiasm. This most commonly presents as a bitemporal hemianopsia (Fig. 4-1).

The gland weighs less than 1 g and is divided into an anterior lobe or adenohypophysis (anterior–adeno) and posterior lobe, or neurohypophysis.

The hormones of the posterior pituitary, vasopressin and oxytocin, are produced in the hypothalamus and are transported to the posterior lobe. Although the anterior pituitary produces its own hormones, prolactin, growth hormone (GH), follicle-stimulating hormone (FSH), luteinizing hormone (LH), adrenocorticotropin (ACTH), and thyrotropin, they are all under the control of hypothalamic hormones that travel directly from the hypothalamus through a portal circulation to the anterior pituitary (Fig. 4-2).

▶ PROLACTINOMA

Pathology

Most prolactin-secreting tumors are not malignant. Prolactin-secreting tumors are divided into macroadenomas and microadenomas. Macroadenomas are characterized by gland enlargement, whereas microadenomas do not cause gland enlargement.

Epidemiology

This is the most common type of pituitary neoplasm. Macroadenomas are more common in men, whereas microadenomas are 10 times more common in women.

History

Macroadenomas usually produce headache as the tumor enlarges. Women may describe irregular menses, amenorrhea, or galactorrhea.

Physical Examination

Defects of extraocular movements occur in 5–10% of patients and reflect compromise of cranial nerves III, IV, or VI. Women may have galactorrhea, whereas only 15% of men will have sexual dysfunction or gynecomastia.

Diagnostic Evaluation

A serum prolactin level of greater than 300 µg/L establishes a diagnosis of pituitary adenoma, whereas a level above 100 µg/L is suggestive. Magnetic resonance imaging (MRI) will differentiate micro- from macroadenomas and allow characterization of local tumor growth.

Treatment

Asymptomatic patients with microadenomas can be followed without treatment. When symptoms of hyperprolactinemia occur, a trial of bromocriptine should be initiated. In the event of failure, transsphenoidal resection provides an 80% short-term cure rate, although long-term relapse may be as high as 40%. For patients who desire children, transsphenoidal resection provides a 40% success for childbearing.

Management options for macroadenomas with compressive symptoms include bromocriptine, which may decrease the size of the tumor, and surgical resection, often in combination. Resection is associated with recurrence rates of 80%. Radiation therapy is effective for long-term control but is associated with panhypopituitarism.

Key Point

1. Prolactinoma is the most common pituitary tumor and is usually not malignant.

▶ GROWTH HORMONE HYPERSECRETION

Pathogenesis

Growth hormone stimulates production of growth-promoting hormones, including somatomedians and insulin-like growth hormone. Overproduction results in acromegaly, which is almost exclusively due to a pituitary adenoma, although abnormalities in hypothalamic production of GH-releasing hormone can also occur.

Epidemiology

Acromegaly has a prevalence of 40 per million.

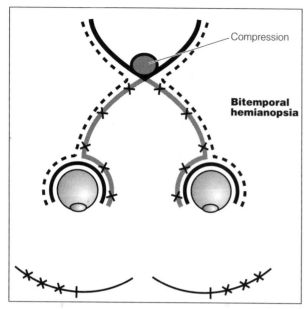

Figure 4-1 Visual disturbances from compressive pituitary lesions.

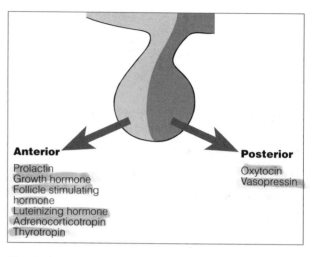

Figure 4-2 Pituitary hormones.

History

Patients may complain of sweating, fatigue, headaches, voice changes, arthralgias, and jaw malocclusion. Symptoms usually develop over a period of years. There may be a history of kidney stones.

Physical Examination

The hallmark of the disease is bony overgrowth of the face and hands with roughened facial features and increased size of the nose, lips, and tongue. Signs of left ventricular hypertrophy occur in over half of all patients and hypertension is common.

Diagnostic Evaluation

Serum GH levels are elevated, and GH is not suppressed by insulin challenge. Insulin resistance may be present. MRI should be obtained to delineate the extent of the lesion.

Treatment

Options include resection, radiation, and bromocriptine. Surgical cure rates are approximately 75% in patient with lower preoperative GH levels but only 35% in patients with high preoperative GH levels. Radiation is effective but slow and may result in panhypopituitarism. Bromocriptine can suppress GH production in combination with other treatment modalities; it is not usually effective as a single therapy.

Key Points

1. The diagnosis of acromegaly is based on characteristic appearance and elevated GH levels.
2. Treatment options include surgery, radiation, and bromocriptine.

▶ FSH AND LH HYPERSECRETION

Epidemiology

These tumors comprise approximately 4% of all pituitary adenomas.

History

Patients usually complain of headache or visual field changes from compression. Symptoms of panhypopituitarism may be preset as the tumors often grow to large size. In the female, there are no symptoms attributable to oversecretion of FSH or LH. Men with FSH-secreting tumors may complain of depressed libido.

Physical Examination

There may be signs of compression.

Diagnostic Evaluation

Hormone levels will be elevated.

Treatment

Surgery is necessary to relieve compression.

▶ THYROTROPIN AND ACTH EXCESS

These diseases are discussed in their respective sections.

▶ ADRENAL

Anatomy and Physiology

The adrenal glands lie just above the kidneys and anterior to the posterior portion of the diaphragm. The right gland is lateral and just posterior to the inferior vena cava and medial to the liver, whereas the left gland is inferior to the stomach and above the pancreas. The blood supply derives from the superior supraadrenal, the middle supraadrenal, and the inferior supraadrenal coming from the inferior phrenic, the aorta, and the renal, respectively. Venous drainage on the right is to the inferior vena cava and to the left is to the renal vein.

The gland is divided into cortex and medulla. The cortex secretes glucocorticoids (cortisol), mineralocorticoids (aldosterone), and sex steroids, whereas the medulla secretes catecholamines (epinephrine, norepinephrine, and dopamine) (Fig. 4-3). Cholesterol is the precursor for both glucocorticoids and mineralocorticoids through a variety of pathways beginning with the formation of pregnenolone, the rate-limiting step for corticoid synthesis.

Cortisol is secreted in response to ACTH from the pituitary, which is in turn controlled by corticotropin releasing factor (CRF) secretion from the hypothalamus. Hypovolemia, hypoxia, hypothermia, and hypoglycemia stimulate cortisol production. Cortisol has many actions, including stimulation of glucagon release and inhibition of insulin release.

Exogenous glucocorticoids suppress the immune system and impair wound healing. They block inflammatory cell migration and inhibit antibody production, histamine release, collagen formation, and fibroblast function. These effects are significant sources of morbidity in patients maintained on steroid therapy.

Figure 4-3 Adrenal hormones.

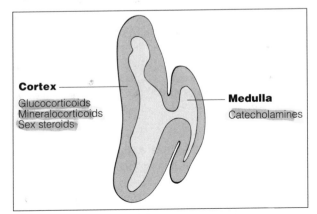

Cortex
Glucocorticoids
Mineralocorticoids
Sex steroids

Medulla
Catecholamines

Aldosterone secretion is controlled by the renin-angiotensin system. In response to decreased renal blood flow or hyponatremia, juxtaglomerular cells secrete renin. This causes cleavage of angiotensinogen to angiotensin I, which in turn is cleaved to angiotensin II. Angiotensin II causes vasoconstriction and stimulates aldosterone secretion. Aldosterone stimulates the distal tubule to reabsorb sodium. This increases water retention and works to restore circulating blood volume and pressure.

Cushing's Syndrome

Pathogenesis

Cushing's syndrome is due to overproduction of cortisol. This occurs secondary to ACTH hypersecretion in approximately 80% of patients. A pituitary adenoma is the cause in 80% of these patients (strictly termed Cushing's *disease*), whereas the remainder derives from other tumors, including small cell carcinoma of the lung and carcinoid tumors of the bronchi and gut. Adrenal adenoma is the cause of cortisol hypersecretion in 10–20% of patients, whereas adrenal carcinoma and excess CRF production from the hypothalamus are unusual sources for increased cortisol production.

History

Patients may complain of weight gain, easy bruising, lethargy, and weakness.

Physical Examination

Patients have a typical appearance with truncal obesity, striae, and hirsutism. Hypertension, proximal muscle weakness, impotence or amenorrhea, osteoporosis, glucose intolerance, and ankle edema may be present.

Diagnostic Evaluation

Increased cortisol production is most reliably demonstrated by 24-hour urine collection. Low ACTH levels suggest an adrenal source, as the autonomously secreted cortisol suppresses ACTH production. The dexamethasone suppression test is useful in differentiating between pituitary microadenomas, macroadenomas, and ectopic sources of ACTH. Dexamethasone is a potent inhibitor of ACTH release. In patients with pituitary microadenomas, dexamethasone is able to suppress ACTH production, whereas in the other patient groups this effect is not seen. Response to CRH stimulation is accentuated when the source is pituitary; there is no response from adrenal or ectopic causes.

Treatment

Therapy is directed toward removing the source of increased cortisol production. For pituitary sources, resection is preferred. For adrenal source, adrenalectomy is curative if the lesion is an adenoma. Resection should be attempted for adrenal carcinoma.

Key Point

1. Cushing's syndrome results from overproduction of cortisol, most commonly due to ACTH overproduction from a pituitary tumor.

Hyperaldosteronism

Pathogenesis

Causes of excess secretion of aldosterone include adrenal adenoma (80%), idiopathic bilateral hyperplasia (15%), adrenal carcinoma (rare), or ectopic production (rare).

Epidemiology

The prevalence among patients with diastolic hypertension is 1 in 200.

History

Symptoms are usually mild and include fatigue and nocturia.

Physical Examination

Hypertension is the most common finding.

Diagnostic Evaluation

Hypokalemia occurs as sodium is preferentially reabsorbed in the distal tubule causing kaliuresis. Aldosterone levels in serum and urine will be increased, and serum renin levels will be decreased. After demonstration of hyperaldosteronism, CT or MRI is used to evaluate the adrenals. The presence of a unilateral adrenal mass greater than 1 cm strongly suggests the diagnosis of adrenal neoplasm.

Treatment

Surgical excision is indicated for adenoma, whereas excision and/or debulking with chemotherapy including cisplatin or mitotane is the treatment of choice for carcinoma. Pharmacologic therapy for patients with idiopathic bilateral hyperplasia usually includes a trial of potassium sparing diuretics and dexamethasone.

Key Point

1. Adrenal adenoma is the most common cause of hyperaldosteronism.

Excess Sex Steroid Production

Adrenal neoplasms can secrete excess sex steroids. Virilization suggests the lesion is malignant. Treatment is surgical removal.

Adrenal Insufficiency

Pathogenesis

Long-term steroid use can lead to suppression of the adrenal cortex. In the setting of surgical stress, the cortex may not be able to respond with the appropriate release of glucocorticoids and mineralocorticoids. These patients are at risk for Addison's disease or acute adrenal insufficiency, which is life threatening.

History

Patients complain of abdominal pain and vomiting.

Physical Examination

Obtundation may occur. Hypotension, hypovolemia, and hyperkalemia can lead to shock and cardiac arrhythmias.

Treatment

Preoperative identification of patients at risk for adrenal suppression is critical, and perioperative steroids are necessary. They should be continued if the patient is in critical condition.

Key Point

1. Patients on steroids preoperatively must be identified and perioperative steroids considered to avoid life-threatening adrenal insufficiency.

Pheochromocytoma

Pathophysiology

This tumor produces an excess of catecholamines.

Epidemiology

This tumor is rare. It occurs most commonly in the third and fourth decades with a slight female predominance. Approximately 5–10% occur in association with syndromes including the multiple endocrine neoplasias types IIa and IIb. Approximately 10% are malignant. Pheochromocytoma is the etiology of hypertension in less than 0.2% of patients. The catecholamine source is most commonly the adrenals but can occur elsewhere in the abdomen (10%) or outside the abdomen (2%).

History

Patients may complain of headaches, tachycardia or palpitations, anxiety, sweating, chest or abdominal pain, and nausea either in paroxysms or constant in nature. Physical exertion, tyramine containing foods, nicotine, succinylcholine, and propranolol can precipitate attacks.

Diagnostic Evaluation

Diagnosis is established by elevated urinary epinephrine and norepinephrine, as well as their metabolites metanephrine, normetanephrine, and vanillylmandelic acid. CT or MRI will yield information about tumor size and location. Nuclear medicine scan using radioactive metaiodobenzylguanidine is especially useful for finding extraadrenal tumors.

Treatment

Pheochromocytomas are removed surgically. Preoperative preparation is critical to assure the patient does not have a hypertensive crisis in the operating room. Alpha blockade with phenoxybenzamine or phentolamine is usually combined with beta blockade. It is important to establish alpha blockade first because in the setting of catecholamine surge, beta blockade will prevent tachycardia in the presence of increased systemic vascular resistance, which can lead to decreased cardiac output and shock.

Key Point

1. Pheochromocytoma may present with paroxysms of headache, flushing, and anxiety. Diagnosis is made on urine examination for catecholamines and catecholamine metabolites.

Multiple Endocrine Neoplasias

MEN I consists of the 3 p's: parathyroid hyperplasia, pancreatic islet cell tumors, and anterior pituitary adenomas. Parathyroid hyperplasia occurs in 90%. Pancreatic neoplasms occur in 50%. These are most commonly gastrinoma, but tumors of cells producing insulin, glucagon, somatostatin, and vasoactive intestinal peptide can also occur. The anterior pituitary tumor is most commonly prolactin secreting and occurs in approximately 25% of patients. MEN IIa consists of medullary thyroid carcinoma, pheochromocytoma, and parathyroid hyperplasia. Medullary thyroid carcinoma (MTC) occurs in almost all affected patients. MEN IIb consists of medullary thyroid carcinoma, pheochromocytoma, and mucosal neuromas with characteristic body habitus including thick lips, kyphosis, and pectus excavatum. Diagnosis and treatment follows treatment for the individual lesion (Fig. 4-4).

Key Points

1. MEN I consists of parathyroid hyperplasia, pancreatic islet cell tumors, and anterior pituitary adenomas.

2. MEN IIa consists of MTC, pheochromocytoma, and parathyroid hyperplasia.

3. MEN IIb consists of MTC, pheochromocytoma, and mucosal neuromas.

Figure 4-4 Multiple endocrine neoplasias.

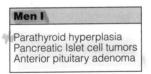

Men I
Parathyroid hyperplasia
Pancreatic Islet cell tumors
Anterior pituitary adenoma

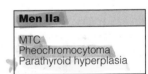

Men IIa
MTC
Pheochromocytoma
Parathyroid hyperplasia

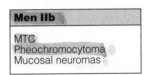

Men IIb
MTC
Pheochromocytoma
Mucosal neuromas

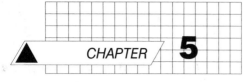

CHAPTER 5

Esophagus

▶ ANATOMY AND PHYSIOLOGY

The esophagus extends from the pharynx to the stomach, bounded posteriorly by the vertebral column and thoracic duct, anteriorly by the trachea, laterally by the pleura, and on the left by the aorta. It courses downward to the left, then to the right, and back to the left to join the stomach. The vagus nerve forms a plexus around the esophagus, which condense to form two trunks on the lateral esophagus. These in turn rotate so that the left trunk moves anteriorly while the right trunk moves posteriorly. The esophageal mucosa is lined by squamous epithelium that becomes columnar near the gastroesophageal junction. The next layer encountered moving radially outward is the submucosa, which contains Meissner's plexus. Next are two muscular layers separated by Auerbach's plexus. There is no true serosa. The superior and inferior thyroid arteries supply the upper esophagus, whereas the intercostals, left gastric, and phrenic arteries supply the lower esophagus. Venous drainage of the upper esophagus is into the inferior thyroid and vertebrals, whereas the mid and lower esophagus drains into the azygous, hemiazygous, and let gastric veins. Submucosal veins can become engorged in patients with portal hypertension, causing varices and bleeding. Lymphatics drain into cervical, mediastinal, celiac, and gastric nodes. Innervation is from the vagus, cervical sympathetic ganglion, splanchnic, and celiac ganglion. These are responsible for esophageal motility.

Peristaltic conveyance of food is mediated by smooth muscle. Gastric reflux is prevented by increased tone in the lower portion of the esophagus; there is no true sphincter. Air ingestion is prevented by resting tone in the upper esophagus.

▶ ESOPHAGEAL NEOPLASMS

Pathology

Esophageal neoplasms are benign in less than 1% of cases. Most cancers are squamous cell, but the incidence of adenocarcinoma is increasing. Benign lesions include leiomyomas and hemangiomas.

Pathogenesis

Factors identified in the development of esophageal cancer include mucosal insult, as occurs in chronic ingestion of extremely hot liquids, esophageal burns from acid or base ingestions, radiation-induced esophagitis, and reflux esophagitis, especially when it results in Barrett's esophagus which occurs when the normal squamous epithelium becomes columnar in response to injury. Alcohol, cigarettes, nitrosamines, and malnutrition have also been implicated. There also is a higher incidence of esophageal cancer in patients with Plummer-Vinson syndrome.

Epidemiology

The incidence of esophageal cancer varies according to the local customs involving the etiologic factors described above. For example, in places with high soil nitrosamine content, the prevalence of esophageal cancer is almost 1% of adults. In the United States, the incidence of esophageal cancer is 4 in 100,000 white males and 12 in 100,000 black males. It is most commonly a disease of men between 50 and 70 years of age.

History

Patients with esophageal cancer usually present with chest pain that is constant in nature or occurs during or after meals. Dysphagia, weight loss, and odynophagia are common.

Physical Examination

Signs are nonspecific and include weight loss or lymphadenopathy.

Diagnostic Evaluation

Esophagogram can detect lesions of less than 1 cm, whereas esophagoscopy with washings and biopsy of strictures will provide a diagnosis in 95% of patients. Esophagoscopy will also define the extent of tumor. Because there is no serosa, disease is often locally invasive on presentation.

Treatment

For local disease, esophagectomy provides possibility of cure. For advanced disease, esophagectomy provides excellent palliation. Esophageal stents are considered in patients who are poor operative candidates, but the incidence of stent complications including esophageal perforation is quite high. Radiation may also be useful for palliation in squamous cell tumors.

Key Points

1. The esophagus lacks a true serosa, so that cancer is often not contained at the time of diagnosis.
2. Most esophageal tumors are malignant.
3. Risk factors for esophageal cancer include Barrett's esophagus, burns, and nitrosamines.

▶ ACHALASIA
Pathophysiology
Achalasia results from absence of peristalsis and failure of the lower esophageal sphincter to relax with swallowing. The cause of this seems to reside in Auerbach's plexus, but the exact mechanism is not well understood.

Epidemiology
Achalasia is the most common esophageal motility disorder, with an incidence 6 per 100,000. Men and women are equally affected. Patients usually present in the fourth through sixth decades.

History
Patients complain of dysphagia. As the column of food or liquid rises in the esophagus, change to a recumbent position may cause liquid to spill into the mouth or into the lungs, and patients may complain of regurgitation or have a history of pneumonia. Because the regurgitant does not include gastric contents, it is not sour tasting.

Diagnostic Evaluation
Esophagogram will demonstrate distal narrowing. Video imaging will reveal abnormal peristalsis. The lower portion of the esophagus may form a bird's beak, and there may be proximal dilation. Motility and pressure studies confirm the diagnosis. Esophagoscopy should also be performed to rule out cancer and evaluate for strictures.

Treatment
Options include balloon dilation of the lower esophageal sphincter or esophagomyotomy, which consists of longitudinal lateral incisions through the esophageal musculature. Both have high rates of success; balloon dilation requires multiple procedures and there is

a risk of rupture. Surgery requires a thoracotomy or thoracoscopy but provides a long-term solution.

Key Points
Achalasia

1. Is the most common disorder of esophageal motility;
2. Can usually be differentiated from cancer by esophagoscopy, but complete evaluation for malignancy should be undertaken.

▶ PERFORATION
Etiology
Esophageal perforation occurs must commonly after instrumentation but can also be due to foreign bodies, trauma, or vigorous vomiting (Boerhaave's esophagus).

History
Recent vomiting or instrumentation is common. The patient may complain of pain at the level of the tear.

Physical Examination
Fever, tachycardia, and circulatory collapse can occur quickly. Mediastinal emphysema may be present. If the rupture violates the pleura, pneumothorax can occur with decreased breath sounds and hypoxia. A crunching sound with each heart beat is occasionally present.

Diagnostic Evaluation
Chest x-ray will demonstrate mediastinal air or pneumothorax. A water-soluble contrast study should be performed to locate the level of the perforation.

Treatment
Thoracotomy, repair of the perforation, and drainage is necessary in most cases. Small cervical lacerations can be managed with antibiotics alone. The mortality due to esophageal perforation is over 50% if any injury to the thoracic esophagus is not treated within 24 hours.

Key Point
Esophageal perforation

1. Is frequently fatal if not diagnosed and treated early.

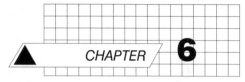

Gallbladder

▶ ANATOMY AND PHYSIOLOGY

The gallbladder is located in the right upper quadrant of the abdomen beneath the liver. The cystic duct exits at the neck of the gallbladder and joins the common hepatic duct to form the common bile duct, which empties into the duodenum at the ampulla of Vater. This is surrounded by the sphincter of Oddi, which regulates bile flow into the duodenum (Fig. 6-1). Bile produced in the liver is stored in the gallbladder. Cholecystokinin stimulates gallbladder contraction and release of bile into the duodenum. The spiral valves of Heister prevent bile reflux back into the gallbladder. Arterial supply is from the cystic artery, which most commonly arises from the right hepatic artery and courses through the triangle of Calot, bounded by the cystic duct, the common hepatic duct, and the edge of the liver.

▶ GALLSTONE DISEASE

Cholelithiasis is the presence of gallstones. Biliary colic is pain produced when the gallbladder contracts against a stone in the neck of the gallbladder or as a stone passes through the bile ducts. Acute cholecystitis refers to infection of the gallbladder; total or partial occlusion of the cystic duct is thought to be required. The most common organisms cultured during an episode of acute cholecystitis are *Escherichia coli, Klebsiella, enterococci, Bacteroides fragilis,* and pseudomonas. Choledocholithiasis refers to stones in the common bile duct (Fig. 6-2).

Figure 6-1 Gallbladder and biliary anatomy.

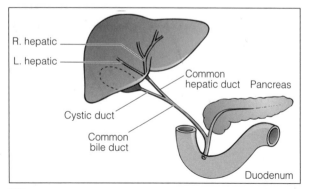

Pathogenesis

Stones can be composed of cholesterol, calcium bilirubinate, or both. Cholesterol stones comprise approximately 80% of all stones in Western countries. Stone formation occurs when bile becomes supersaturated with cholesterol. Stones then precipitate out of solution. High cholesterol diet causes increased concentrations of cholesterol and probably has a role in the pathogenesis of cholesterol stones. Calcium bilirubinate (pigment stones) are found in association with hemolytic processes, chronic biliary infection, and cirrhosis.

Epidemiology

Approximately 10% of the population of the United States has gallstones. They are more common in women; other risk factors include obesity, multiparity, diabetes, and age over the fifth decade. Gallstones are an important cause of pancreatitis.

History

Most patients with stones are asymptomatic. Patients with biliary colic usually complain of right upper quadrant pain, but the pain may be epigastric. It commonly occurs after eating and may be precipitated by fatty meals. Unlike peptic ulcer disease, biliary colic is exacerbated by oral intake. Nausea and vomiting may be present. A typical episode may last on the order of hours. Cholecystitis implies infection, and these patients may complain of pain that is longer lasting, shaking chills, and severe vomiting. Patients with choledocholithiasis may relate clay colored stools or dark urine caused by inability of bile pigments to reach the stool and subsequent reflux into the bloodstream and renal clearance into the urine. Patients with cholangitis also complain of right upper quadrant pain, and fever or chills may be present. Pancreatitis typically manifests with epigastric pain radiating to the back, constant in nature and of longer duration.

Physical Examination

Physical examination in simple biliary colic will reveal right upper quadrant tenderness but usually no fever. Cholecystitis may be associated with fever and signs of peritoneal irritation including right upper quadrant rebound and guarding. Right upper quadrant tenderness

Gallstone Pancreatitis
↑ Amylase
↑ Lipase

Cholangitis   Charcot's triad
Fever
RUQ Pain
Jaundice

Raynaud's Pentad
Hypotension
MS Δ's

Gallbladder ▼23

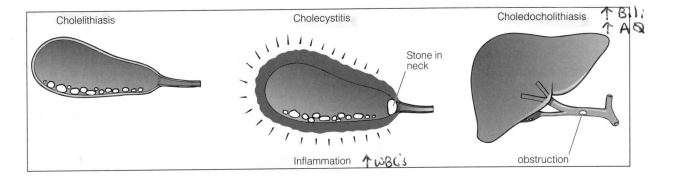

Figure 6-2 Biliary pathology.

may cause a sudden arrest of inspiratory effort as the examiner's hand contacts the inflamed gall bladder. This is known as Murphy's sign. Choledocholithiasis may be associated with jaundice in addition to signs of biliary colic. Cholangitis is marked by Charcot's triad of fever, right upper quadrant pain, and jaundice. Progression of this to sepsis defines the Raynaud's pentad by adding hypotension and mental status changes. Patients who have developed gallstone pancreatitis will exhibit severe epigastric tenderness.

Diagnostic Evaluation

Laboratory examination in biliary colic is often unremarkable. Cholecystitis usually manifests with increased white blood cell count. Choledocholithiasis is associated with increased bilirubin and alkaline phosphatase. Cholangitis will usually have elevated bilirubin and transaminase levels. Gallstone pancreatitis is accompanied by elevations in serum amylase and lipase.

Ultrasound has a sensitivity and specificity of 98% for gallstones. The stones present as an opacity with an echoless shadow posteriorly (Fig. 6-3). Moving the patient will demonstrate migration of the stones to the dependent portion of the gallbladder. Ultrasound can also be used to detect acute cholecystitis. Fluid around the gallbladder, a thickened gallbladder wall, and gallbladder distention all support the diagnosis of acute cholecystitis. Ultrasound is not accurate for common duct stones. Cholescintigraphy is almost 100% sensitive and 95% specific for acute cholecystitis. In this test, a radionucleotide is injected intravenously. It is taken up in the liver and excreted into the biliary tree. If the cystic duct is obstructed, as in acute cholecystitis, the gallbladder will not fill, and the radionucleotide will pass directly into the duodenum. Endoscopic retrograde cholangiopancreatography is performed by visualizing the ampulla where the pancreatic and biliary ducts enter the duodenum. Contrast is passed retrograde and outlines the biliary tree and pancreatic ducts. This technique is useful for identifying common duct stones in patients in whom choledocholithiasis or pancreatitis is suspected. KUB will show 20% of gallstones.

Complications

Pancreatitis may occur as a common duct stone passes through the ampulla and bile refluxes into the pancreatic ducts. Emphysematous cholecystitis occurs most commonly in diabetics and is due to clostridium perfringens. Perforation occurs in approximately 5% of cases. A large stone may cause a fistula between the gallbladder and bowel; passage of a large stone through this fistula may cause gallstone ileus.

Treatment

For patients with asymptomatic stones found on workup for other problems, the incidence of symptoms or complications is approximately 2% per year. Cholecystectomy is generally not advised for these patients.

Figure 6-3 Gallbladder ultrasound—cholethiasis.

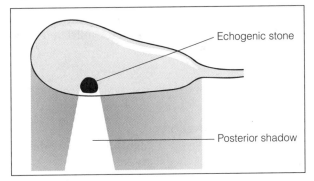

For patients with biliary colic laparoscopic cholecystectomy is a safe and effective procedure. This is ideally done in an elective setting, after the patient's symptoms resolve. If the preoperative workup suggests that common duct stones may be present, either endoscopic retrograde cholangiopancreatography (ERCP) or intraoperative cholangiogram should be considered.

Patients with acute cholecystitis should be resuscitated with fluids because vomiting and infection are likely to have caused dehydration. Broad-spectrum intravenous antibiotics (e.g., ampicillin, gentamycin, and flagyl) should be started, and nasogastric suction should be initiated. In all but the sickest patients, the gallbladder should be removed on a semiurgent basis. Laparoscopic cholecystectomy is considered safe but tends to be more difficult and associated with a higher rate of conversion to open cholecystectomy when done within a few days of an episode of cholecystitis. For patients too sick to tolerate cholecystectomy, a cholecystostomy tube should be considered. This is a relatively simple procedure that involves placing a drain into the gallbladder to decompress and drain the infection. It may be placed percutaneously or under direct vision in the operating room. Cholecystectomy is then carried out at a later date.

Patients with gallstone pancreatitis are fluid resuscitated and placed on nasogastric suction. The role of antibiotics is unclear. The value of early ERCP with sphincterotomy in acute attacks is controversial. Early cholecystectomy is advocated because the risk of recurrent pancreatitis is approximately 40% within 6 weeks. At the time of operation, intraoperative cholangiogram with common duct exploration if stones are present is advocated to remove residual stones.

Cholangitis on the basis of choledocholithiasis is managed with broad-spectrum antibiotics, nasogastric suction, and fluid resuscitation. For patients who do not improve, ERCP with sphincterotomy is necessary to decompress bile ducts. Decompression can also be accomplished by an open surgical procedure, but carries a high mortality in these sick patients.

Key Points

1. Cholelithiasis refers to stones in the gallbladder, typically symptoms include right upper quadrant pain.
2. Cholecystitis implies infection in the gallbladder, typically symptoms include right upper quadrant pain and sign of infection.
3. Choledocholithiasis refers to stones in the common bile duct, and patients will often have increased bilirubin.
4. Cholangitis refers to infection in the small duct of the liver, and patients will often have right upper quadrant pain, fever, and jaundice.
5. Pancreatitis is an important complication of gallstone disease.

▶ CANCER OF THE GALLBLADDER

Epidemiology

Cancer of the gallbladder is three times more common in females. The incidence is 2.5 in 100,000. Risk factors include gallstones, porcelain gallbladder, and adenoma. Large gallstones carry greater risk.

Pathology

Approximately 80% are adenocarcinomas, 10% are anaplastic, and 5% are squamous.

History

Patients usually present with vague right upper quadrant pain. Weight loss and anorexia may also be present.

Physical Examination

There may be right upper quadrant mass. Jaundice represents invasion of compression of the biliary system.

Treatment

Options include radical resection of the gallbladder, including partial hepatic resection, or palliative operation as symptoms arise.

Prognosis

Unless the cancer is found incidentally at cholecystectomy for stones, only 4% of patients will be alive in 5 years.

▶ BILE DUCT CANCERS

Epidemiology

These cancers are rare. Risk factors include ulcerative colitis, sclerosing cholangitis, and infection with *Clonorchis sinensis*.

History

Patients with advanced disease typically complain of right upper quadrant pain.

Physical Examination

There may be a distended gallbladder or jaundice as the tumor obstructs the biliary tree.

Diagnostic Evaluation

Ultrasound and computed tomography will show evidence of obstruction, but percutaneous transhepatic cholangiography (PTC) or ERCP is usually necessary to demonstrate the lesion.

Treatment

Treatment consists of surgical resection.

Prognosis

Mortality is 90% at 5 years.

Key Point

1. Gallbladder and bile duct cancers are rare and usually fatal.

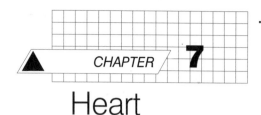

CHAPTER 7

Heart

► ANATOMY

Coronary circulation begins at the sinus of valsalva where the right and left coronary arteries (RCA, LCA) arise. The left main (LM) artery branches into the left anterior descending (LAD) and the left circumflex (LCX) arteries. The LAD supplies the anterior of the left ventricle as well as the apex of the heart, the intraventricular septum, and the portion of the right ventricle that borders the intraventricular septum. The LCX travels in the groove separating the left atrium and ventricle and gives off marginal branches to the left ventricle. The RCA travels between the right atrium and ventricle to supply the lateral portion of the right ventricle (Fig. 7-1). The posterior descending artery (PDA) comes from the RCA in 90% of patients and supplies the atriovenous node. Patients whose PDA arises from the RCA are termed right dominant. If the PDA arises from the left circumflex, the system is left dominant.

The aortic valve is located between the left ventricle and the aorta. It usually has three leaflets. The sinuses formed at the base of each leaflet give rise to the RCA and LCA, with the third leaflet forming the noncoronary sinus. The mitral valve is located between the left atrium and ventricle. It normally has two leaflets, the anterior protruding further across the valve. Chordae tendinae attach the leaflets to the papillary muscles, which in turn serve to tether the leaflets to the ventricular wall.

► CORONARY ARTERY DISEASE (CAD)

Epidemiology

Atherosclerosis of the coronary arteries is the most common cause of mortality in the United States, responsible for one third of all deaths. Approximately five million Americans have CAD. The disease is five times more prevalent in males than females. Risk factors include hypertension, family history, hypercholesterolemia, smoking, obesity, diabetes, and physical inactivity.

Pathophysiology

Coronary artery stenosis is a gradual process that begins in the second decade. When the lumen decreases to 75% of the native area, the lesion becomes hemodynamically significant.

History

Patients with ischemic heart disease usually complain of substernal chest pain or pressure that may radiate down the arms or into the jaw, teeth, or back. Typically the pain will occur during periods of physical exertion or emotional stress. Episodes that resolve with rest are termed stable angina. If the pain occurs at rest or does not improve with rest, is new and severe, or is progressive it is termed unstable angina and suggests impending infarction.

Physical Examination

There may be evidence of peripheral vascular disease including diminished pulses. Signs of ventricular failure including cardiomegaly, congestive heart failure, an S3 or S4, or murmur of mitral regurgitation may occur.

Diagnostic Evaluation

The electrocardiogram (ECG) may show signs of ischemia or an old infarct. A chest radiograph may show an enlarged heart or pulmonary congestion. An exercise stress test is sensitive in identifying myocardium at risk. These areas can be localized using nuclear medicine scans including thallium imaging. Echocardiography is extremely useful in evaluating myocardial function and valvular competence. Angiography is the gold standard for identifying lesions in the coronary arteries, assessing their severity, and planning operative intervention.

Treatment

Patients with severe disease of the LM or with severe disease in the three major coronary arteries have decreased mortality after coronary artery bypass surgery. Pain is reliably relieved in over 85% of patients. Surgical options include bypass using the internal mammary arteries or saphenous veins. Internal mammary bypass is preferred because of higher patency rates.

Key Points

Coronary artery disease

1. Is the leading cause of mortality in the United States;

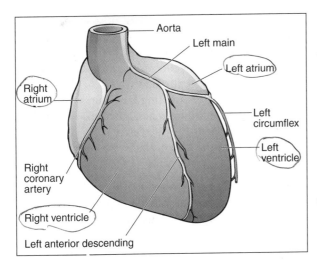

Figure 7-1 Coronary anatomy.

2. Has risk factors that include hypertension, smoking, obesity, diabetes, hypercholesterolemia, inactivity, and family history;

3. Is treated surgically if all three coronary arteries or left main coronary artery are diseased, or if patients have debilitating symptoms.

▶ AORTIC STENOSIS (AS)

Etiology
AS can present congenitally, for example when the valve is unicuspid, but more commonly occurs in the older population. A congenitally bicuspid valve usually causes aortic stenosis by the time the patient reaches 70 years of age. Other causes include rheumatic fever, which results in commissural fusion and subsequent calcification, and degenerative stenosis in which calcification occurs in the native valve.

Pathophysiology
The initial physiologic response to aortic stenosis is left ventricular hypertrophy to preserve stroke volume and cardiac output. Left ventricular hypertrophy and increasing resistance at the level of the valve result in decreased cardiac output, pulmonary hypertension, and myocardial ischemia.

History
Patients often complain of angina, syncope, and dyspnea, with dyspnea being the worst prognostic indicator.

Physical Examination
There may be a midsystolic ejection murmur as well as cardiomegaly and other signs of congestive heart fail-

ure. Pulsus parvis et tardis, a delayed, diminish impulse at the carotid, may be appreciated.

Diagnostic Evaluation
Echocardiography or cardiac catheterization reliably studies the valve. A decrease in the aortic valve area from the normal 3 or 4 cm to less than 1 cm signifies severe disease.

Treatment
Patients who are symptomatic should undergo aortic valve replacement unless other medical conditions make it unlikely the patient could survive the operation. In asymptomatic individuals, progressive cardiomegaly is an indication for operation, as surgical therapy is superior to medical therapy.

Key Points
Aortic stenosis

1. Can be caused by a congenital bicuspid valve or rheumatic fever;

2. Symptoms include angina, syncope, and dyspnea.

▶ AORTIC INSUFFICIENCY (AI)

Etiology
AI can be caused by rheumatic fever, connective tissue disorders including Marfan's and Ehlers-Danlos, endocarditis, aortic dissection, and trauma.

Pathophysiology
The incompetent valve causes a decrease in cardiac output and left ventricular dilatation occurs. The larger ventricle is subject to higher wall stress, which increases myocardial oxygen demand.

History
Patients will complain of angina or symptoms of systolic dysfunction.

Physical Examination
Typically, there is a crescendo-decrescendo diastolic murmur and a wide pulse pressure with a water hammer quality. The PMI may be displaced or diffuse.

Diagnostic Evaluation
Echocardiography is a sensitive and specific means of making the diagnosis.

Treatment
Symptomatic patients should undergo replacement if their medical condition allows them to tolerate a major procedure.

Key Points

Aortic regurgitation

1. Can be caused by rheumatic fever, endocarditis, connective tissue disorders, aortic dissection, and trauma;

2. Symptoms include angina and dyspnea.

▶ MITRAL STENOSIS (MS)

Etiology

The overwhelming cause is rheumatic heart disease, as 40% of patients with rheumatic heart disease will develop MS. Rheumatic heart disease occurs after pharyngitis caused by group A streptococcus. A likely autoimmune phenomenon causes a pancarditis resulting in fibrosis of valve leaflets. Histologic findings include Aschoff's nodules. MS may also be due to malignant carcinoid and systemic lupus erythematosus.

Pathophysiology

Fibrosis progresses over a period of two or three decades, causing fusion of the leaflets, which take on a characteristic fish-mouth appearance, significantly impeding blood flow through the valve. Increased left atrial pressures lead to left atrial hypertrophy, which in turn may cause atrial fibrillation or pulmonary hypertension. The pulmonary hypertension can further progress to right ventricular hypertrophy and right heart failure.

Epidemiology

MS has a female predominance of 2:1.

History

Characteristic complaints include dyspnea and fatigability. Occasionally, pulmonary hypertension may lead to hemoptysis.

Physical Examination

There may be cachexia or symptoms of congestive heart failure with pulmonary rales and tachypnea. Jugular venous distention, peripheral edema, ascites, and a sternal heave of right ventricular hypertrophy may be appreciated. Heart sounds are usually characteristic and consist of an opening snap followed by a low rumbling murmur. The splitting of the second heart sound is decreased, and the pulmonary component is louder. The heart rate may demonstrate the irregularly irregular pattern of atrial fibrillation.

Diagnostic Evaluation

Chest x-ray may show cardiomegaly including signs of left atrial hypertrophy. Pulmonary edema may be ap-

preciable. ECG may show atrial fibrillation. Broad, notched P-waves are an indication of left atrial hypertrophy. Right axis deviation is evidence of right ventricular hypertrophy. Echocardiography with Doppler flow measurement is extremely useful for demonstrating mitral stenosis, estimating flow, and assessing the presence of thrombi. Cardiac catheterization gives a direct measurement of transvalvular pressure gradient, from which the area of the mitral annulus can be calculated.

Therapy

Surgical options include valvulotomy or replacement. Therapy is indicated for symptomatic patients.

Key Points

Mitral stenosis

1. Is most commonly caused by rheumatic fever;

2. Symptoms include fatigue and dyspnea.

▶ MITRAL REGURGITATION (MR)

Etiology

Approximately 40% of cases are due to rheumatic fever; other causes include idiopathic calcification associated with hypertension, diabetes, aortic stenosis, and renal failure. Mitral valve prolapse will progress to MR in 5% of affected individuals. Less common causes include myocardial ischemia, trauma, endocarditis, and hypertrophic cardiomyopathy.

Pathophysiology

As regurgitation becomes hemodynamically significant, the left ventricle dilates to preserve cardiac output. A significant volume is ejected retrograde, increasing cardiac work, left atrial volumes, and increasing pulmonary venous pressure. This in turn may lead to left atrial enlargement and fibrillation or cause pulmonary hypertension which may result in right ventricular failure.

Epidemiology

The disease is more common than MS and has a male predominance.

History

Patients commonly complain of dyspnea, orthopnea, and fatigue.

Physical Examination

Patients may appear cachectic. Frequently, there is an irregular pulse, pulmonary rales, and a sternal heave. The pulse characteristically has a rapid upstroke, and a waves may be present. A holosystolic murmur that radiates to the axilla or back is common. The point of maximal impulse is often displaced.

Diagnostic Evaluation

Chest x-ray may show cardiomegaly and pulmonary edema. ECG commonly demonstrates left ventricular or biventricular hypertrophy, left atrial enlargement, and "P mitral." Echocardiography is extremely useful in establishing the diagnosis and the underlying lesion. Cardiac catheterization is useful to establish pulmonary pressures and cardiac output.

Treatment

Medical therapy consists of afterload reducing agents such as angiotensin converting enzyme (ACE) inhibitors, nitroglycerine, and diuretics. Surgical intervention is indicated if congestive failure interferes with daily life, if pulmonary hypertension or left ventricular dilation worsens, or if atrial fibrillation develops. In patients who develop acute MR from endocarditis, ischemia, or trauma, aggressive treatment with afterload reduction, a balloon pump if necessary, and antibiotics if indicated should be used to convert an emergent operation to an elective one. Because of the severe hemodynamic instability that can occur, operative intervention involving repair or replacement may be necessary in the acute setting. These emergent operations carry greater than 15% mortality.

Key Points

Mitral regurgitation

1. Is caused by rheumatic fever, idiopathic calcification, mitral valve prolapse, myocardial ischemia, trauma, endocarditis, and hypertrophic cardiomyopathy;

2. Symptoms include fatigue and dyspnea.

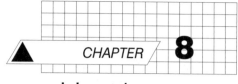

CHAPTER 8

Hernias

A hernia occurs when a defect or weakness in a muscular or fascial layer allows tissue to abnormally protrude. Hernias are divided into reducible, incarcerated, and strangulated. Reducible hernias can be returned to their body cavity of origin. Incarcerated hernias cannot be returned to their body cavity of origin. Strangulated hernias contain tissue with a compromised vascular supply. These are particularly dangerous because they lead to tissue necrosis and, in the case of bowel, can produce obstruction, perforation, sepsis, and death.

▶ EPIDEMIOLOGY

Between 500,000 and 1,000,000 hernia repairs are performed each year. Five percent of people will have an inguinal hernia repair during their lifetime. Half of all hernias are indirect inguinal, and a quarter are direct inguinal. In decreasing incidence are incisional and ventral (10%), femoral (6%), and umbilical (3%). Indirect inguinal hernias are the most common hernia in both males and females; overall, hernias have a 5:1 male predominance. Femoral hernias are more common in females than in males.

▶ INGUINAL HERNIAS
Anatomy

The abdominal contents are kept intraperitoneal by three fascial layers, the external oblique, the internal oblique, and the transversalis. The external oblique inserts onto the pubic tubercle; just lateral to this there is an opening, called the external ring, which allows the spermatic cord to escape down into the scrotum. The external ring has no function in the pathogenesis of hernias. The next innermost layer, the internal oblique, forms the cremaster muscle, which envelops the cord as it descends. The innermost layer, the transversalis fascia, arches to join the pubic tubercle. This arch helps to define the superior aspect of the internal ring. During development, the testes begin in an intraperitoneal position and descend through the internal ring, taking with them a layer of peritoneum that is stretched into a hollow tube called the processus vaginalis. This path taken by the testes could also be taken by the bowel, except two things occur. First, the processus vaginalis collapses from a tube into a cord. Next, the transversalis maintains the integrity of the ring. An indirect inguinal hernia occurs when the processus vaginalis fails to obliterate. In this case, bowel or other abdominal contents can escape from their intraperitoneal location. A direct hernia occurs when the transversalis becomes weakened, allowing abdominal contents to herniate directly through the fascia (Fig. 8-1).

History

Patients with reducible inguinal hernias describe an intermittent bulge in the groin or scrotum. Persistence of the bulge raises concern for incarcerated hernia. Severe pain at the hernia or in the abdomen, nausea, or vomiting may occur if the hernia becomes strangulated.

Physical Examination

A finger is placed at the pubic tubercle and pushed upward to find the internal ring; a bulge or pressure as the patient coughs or bears down may be felt. Reducible hernias can be pushed back into the abdomen, incarcerated hernias cannot, and strangulated hernias will be tender, possibly with abdominal distention or signs of peritoneal irritation, including rebound pain and guarding.

Treatment

Reducible inguinal hernias should be repaired on an elective basis. When a hernia is not reducible with gentle pressure, a trial of Trendelenburg position, sedation, and more forceful pressure should be attempted. It is critical that the reduction not take place if the hernia is thought to be strangulated. Reduction of dead tissue into the abdomen will produce bowel perforation and possible sepsis and death. An incarcerated hernia should be operated on urgently, whereas a strangulated hernia is a surgical emergency.

▶ UMBILICAL HERNIAS

These hernias occur at the umbilicus and are congenital. Most resolve spontaneously by the age of 2.

Epidemiology

The incidence is 10% of whites and 40–90% of blacks.

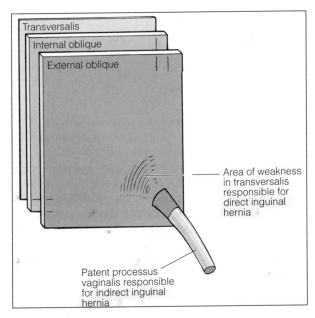

Figure 8-1 Anatomy of inguinal hernias.

History

The patient will relate a bulge at the umbilicus.

Treatment

Indications for operation include incarceration or strangulation or cosmetic concerns. Because large hernias may become incarcerated, they should be repaired.

▶ OTHER HERNIAS

Femoral hernias occur through the femoral canal. Incisional hernias occur through surgical incision, usually as the result of infection. Ventral hernias occur in the midline. Internal hernias are an important cause of bowel obstruction. They occur in patients after abdominal operations when bowel gets trapped due to adhesions or new anatomic relationships. Treatment for all of the above are based on the principles outlined.

Key Points

1. Hernias are extremely common; inguinal are most common and 5% of people will require repair during their lifetime.

2. Inguinal hernias are based on the internal ring.

3. Hernias that become incarcerated should be fixed urgently.

4. Hernias that become strangulated are a surgical emergency.

5. Umbilical hernias are congenital, more common in blacks and frequently resolve spontaneously.

6. Other hernia types include femoral, ventral, incisional, and internal.

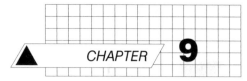

CHAPTER 9

Kidneys and Bladder

► ANATOMY

The kidneys are retroperitoneal structures. They are surrounded by Gerota's fascia and lie lateral to the psoas muscles and inferior to the posterior diaphragm. Blood supply is by renal arteries, which may be paired. The renal veins drain into the inferior vena cava. The ureters course retroperitoneally, in proximity to the cecum on the right and sigmoid colon on the left. They cross the iliac vessels as they enter the true pelvis to empty into the bladder. The bladder lies below the peritoneum in the true pelvis and is covered by a fold of peritoneum. Blood supply is from the iliac arteries through the superior, middle, and inferior vesical arteries. Sympathetic nerve supply is from L1 and L2 roots, whereas parasympathetic is from S2, S3, and S4.

► STONE DISEASE
Etiology

Kidney stones are most commonly calcium phosphate and calcium oxalate (80%); struvite (15%), uric acid (5%), and cystine (1%) are other causes. Calcium stones are most commonly idiopathic but can be caused by hyperuricosuria and hyperparathyroidism. Struvite stones are caused by infection with urease-producing organisms, usually proteus. Uric acid stones are common in patients with gout, and can occur with Lesch-Nyan syndrome or tumors. Cystine stones are hereditary.

Epidemiology

Approximately 20% of males and 10% of females will be affected by nephrolithiasis over their lifetime. Calcium stones and struvite stones are more common in women. Uric acid stones are twice as common in men, and cystine stones occur with equal frequency in men and women.

History

Patients with stone disease usually present with acute onset of pain beginning in the flank and radiating down to the groin, although the pain can be anywhere along this track. The patient is often unable to find a comfortable position, and vomiting is common. Dysuria, frequency, and hematuria may be described.

Diagnostic Evaluation

Workup includes evaluation of urinary sediment that will show hematuria unless the affected ureter is totally obstructed. Crystals will frequently be observed. Calcium oxalate stones are either dumbbell shaped or bipyramidal and may be birefringent. Uric acid crystals are small and red-orange. Cystine stones are flat, hexagonal, and yellow. Struvite stones are rectangular prisms. Abdominal radiograph should be obtained, as calcium, struvite, and cystine stones are all radio-opaque. Intravenous pyelogram involves intravenous administration of an iodinated dye that is excreted in the kidneys. This allows diagnosis of stones by outlining defects in the ureter or demonstrating complete obstruction due to stone disease. Retrograde pyelogram involves injecting dye through the urethra and is useful for assessing the degree and level of obstruction. Ultrasonography of the kidneys can demonstrate hydronephrosis indicative of total ureteral obstruction. The presence of fluid jets at the entrance of the ureter in the bladder precludes the diagnosis of total obstruction.

Treatment

In the acute setting pain and nausea should be controlled with narcotics and anti-emetics. Most stones will pass spontaneously. If the stones are totally obstructing, fail to pass, renal function is deteriorating, or if pain or nausea cannot be controlled, lithotripsy or cystoscopy with stone removal should be considered. Nephrostomy tubes can be placed to decompress the collecting system in the presence of hydronephrosis or infection if obstruction is complete and stone removal is not achieved.

Key Points

Kidney stones

1. Are most commonly composed of calcium salts;
2. Usually present with severe flank pain, which may radiate to the groin;
3. Pass spontaneously in most cases.

▶ RENAL CANCER

Epidemiology

Two percent of cancer deaths are attributable to renal cancer. Males are affected twice as commonly as females, and smoking may be a risk factor.

Pathology

Tumors are divided into granular cell, tubular adenocarcinoma, Wilms' tumor, and sarcoma.

History

Patients may experience hematuria and flank pain that can be sudden in the event of hemorrhage. Fever and extrarenal pain from metastatic disease may be present.

Physical Examination

Tumors may be palpable.

Diagnostic Evaluation

Intravenous pyelogram will demonstrate a defect in the renal silhouette. Computed tomography can differentiate between cystic and solid lesions.

Treatment

Treatment in most cases is radical nephrectomy.

Key Point

Renal cancer

1. Is responsible for 2% of cancer deaths and treatment in most cases is radical nephrectomy.

▶ BLADDER CANCER

Pathology

Transitional cell tumors comprise 90% of bladder malignancies. The remainder are squamous cell and adenocarcinoma.

Epidemiology

Men are three times more frequently affected than women. Smoking, beta-naphthylamine, and paraminodiphenyl all predispose to the development of bladder cancer.

History

Most patients will present with hematuria. Urinary tract infections (UTIs) are relatively common, as is bladder irritability evidenced by frequency and dysuria.

Diagnostic Evaluation

Urinary cytology may reveal the presence of bladder cancer. Cystoscopy with biopsy will confirm the diagnosis. Excretory urography may demonstrate the lesion.

Treatment

For local disease, transurethral resection with chemotherapy including doxorubicin, mitomycin C, or thiotepa is effective. For locally advanced disease, radical cystectomy (including prostatectomy in men) is combined with radiation and chemotherapy.

Key Points

Bladder cancer

1. Usually presents with hematuria.
2. Treatment may be transurethral resection for local disease, whereas radical cystectomy is used for advanced disease.

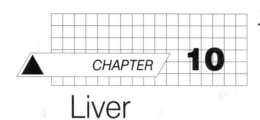

CHAPTER 10

Liver

▶ ANATOMY AND PHYSIOLOGY

The liver is located in the right upper quadrant of the abdomen, bounded superiorly and posteriorly by the diaphragm; laterally by the ribs; and inferiorly by the gallbladder, stomach duodenum, colon, kidney, and right adrenal. It is covered by Glisson's capsule and peritoneum. The falciform ligament between the liver and diaphragm divides the surface of the liver into right and left; this is a landmark between the lateral and medial segments of the left lobe. The coronary ligaments continue laterally from the falciform and end at the right and left triangular ligaments. These ligaments define an area of the liver devoid of peritoneum and termed the bare area of the liver. The liver parenchyma is divided into eight segments based on arterial and venous anatomy (Fig. 10-1).

The hepatic circulation is based on a portal circulation that provides the liver with first access to all intestinal venous flow. Seventy-five percent of total hepatic blood flow is derived from the portal vein, which is formed from the confluence of the splenic and superior mesenteric veins. The remaining blood supply comes from the hepatic artery. Because of this, ligation of the right or left hepatic artery does not usually lead to liver infarction. The hepatic artery usually arises from the celiac axis. The right hepatic artery arises from the superior mesenteric artery in 15% of patients and the left hepatic arises from the left gastric in 15% of patients. Blood leaving the liver enters the inferior vena cava via the right, middle, and left hepatic veins.

The liver is the site of many critical events in energy metabolism. Glucose is taken up and stored as glycogen, and glycogen is broken down as necessary to maintain a relatively constant level of serum glucose. In the fasting state, stored glycogen can meet systemic energy demands for 48 hours. At this point, the liver is able to initiate gluconeogenesis, which converts primarily muscle protein to glucose. In prolonged fasting, the liver contains the enzymes of the Cori cycle to convert products of glucose metabolism (lactate and pyruvate) back into glucose. Additionally, the liver can oxidize fatty acids to ketones, which can be used as an energy source by the brain.

Protein synthetic functions of the liver include the coagulation factors fibrinogen, prothrombin, prekallikrein, high-molecular-weight kininogen, and factors V, VII, VIII, IX, X, XI, and XII. Of these, prothrombin and factors VII, IX, and X are dependent on vitamin K. The anticoagulant coumadin affects these vitamin K-dependent pathways, resulting in an increased prothrombin time. Albumin and alpha globulin are produced solely in the liver.

Digestive functions of the liver include bile synthesis and cholesterol metabolism. Heme, derived from erythrocyte breakdown, is used to form bilirubin, which is taken up in the liver and excreted in the bile after conjugation with glycine or taurine. Bile emulsifies fats to aid their digestion and plays a role in vitamin uptake. Bile salts excreted into the intestine are then reabsorbed in their initial form (most commonly cholic or chenodeoxycholic acid) or after bacterial metabolism to secondary bile salts (most commonly deoxycholic or lithocholic acid). This reabsorption into the portal circulation allows immediate reuptake in the liver without increased systemic concentrations of bile salts. This cycle of bile excretion and absorption is termed the enterohepatic circulation. Total body bile circulates approximately 10 times per day in this loop. Greater than 95% of excreted bile is reabsorbed, and the remainder must be resynthesized. The rate-limiting step of cholesterol synthesis involving the enzyme HMG-CoA reductase occurs in the liver, as does cholesterol metabolism to bile salts.

Detoxification occurs in the liver through two pathways. Phase I reactions involve cytochrome P-450 and include oxidation, reduction, and hydrolysis. Phase II reactions consist of conjugation. These reactions are critical to destruction or renal clearance of toxins. The dosing of all oral drugs is determined only after considering the first pass effect of the drug through the liver. The initial hydroxylation of vitamin D occurs in the liver.

Immunologic functions are mediated by Kupffer's cells, the resident liver macrophages.

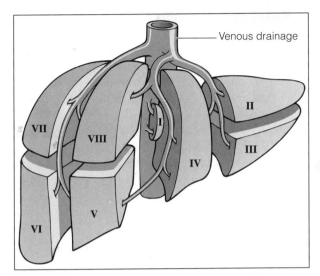

Figure 10-1 Segmental anatomy of the liver.

Key Point

The liver

1. Performs a tremendous array of functions involving energy metabolism, protein synthesis, digestion, and detoxification.

▶ BENIGN LIVER TUMORS

Pathology

These include hepatocellular adenoma, focal nodular hyperplasia, hemangioma, and lipoma. Hemangiomas are divided into capillary and cavernous types, the former being of no clinical consequence and the latter capable of attaining large size and rupturing.

Epidemiology

Only 5% of liver tumors are benign, with hemangioma being the most common. Approximately 7% of people will have a cavernous hemangioma at autopsy. The incidence of adenoma is 1 per million. Oral contraceptive use multiplies this risk by 40. Adenoma and focal nodular hyperplasia are five times more common in females.

History

Adenomas and hemangiomas can be asymptomatic or present with dull pain; rupture can produce sudden onset of severe abdominal pain. These lesions can also become large enough to cause jaundice or symptoms of gastric outlet obstruction, including nausea and vomiting. Focal nodular hyperplasia is rarely symptomatic.

Physical Examination

Large lesions may be palpated. Jaundice may occur in patients if the tumor causes bile duct obstruction.

Diagnostic Evaluation

These lesions are most often found incidentally at laparotomy or on imaging studies requested for other reasons. Laboratory evaluation is often unremarkable, although hemorrhage in an adenoma can lead to hepatocellular necrosis and a subsequent rise in transaminase levels. Hemangioma can cause a consumptive coagulopathy. Computed tomography (CT) is useful for evaluation and operative planning. Adenomas are typically low density lesions; focal nodular hyperplasia may appear as a filling defect or scar, whereas hemangioma will have early peripheral enhancement after contrast administration. Hemangiomas should not be biopsied because of the risk of bleeding.

Treatment

Patients with adenoma who are using oral contraceptives should stop. If the lesion does not regress, resection should be considered in otherwise healthy individuals because of the risk or malignant degeneration or hemorrhage. Relative contraindications to resection include a tumor that is technically difficult to resect or tumors of large size in which a large portion of the liver would need to be removed. Symptomatic hemangiomas should be resected if possible. Because focal nodular hyperplasia is not malignant and rarely causes symptoms, it should not be resected unless it is found incidentally at laparotomy and is small and peripheral enough to be wedged out easily.

Key Point

1. Only 5% of liver tumors are benign.

▶ LIVER CANCER

Pathology

Liver cancers are hepatomas, also known as hepatocellular carcinoma, or metastases from other primaries.

Epidemiology

Ninety-five percent of liver tumors are malignant. Hepatoma is one of the most common malignancy in the world, but rates in the United States are relatively low, approximately 2 per 100,000. It is more common in males than in females.

Etiology

Cirrhosis is a predisposing factor to hepatoma; as such hepatitis B, the leading cause of cirrhosis, and alcoholism are associated with hepatoma development. It is unclear if hepatoma is an end point of hepatocellular damage or caused directly by the virus. Fungal derived aflatoxins have been implicated as causes of hepatoma, as has hemochromatosis, smoking, vinyl chloride, and oral contraceptives.

History

Patients with hepatoma may complain of weight loss, right upper quadrant or shoulder pain, and weakness. Hepatic metastases are often indistinguishable from primary hepatocellular carcinoma.

Physical Examination

Hepatomegaly may be appreciated, and signs of portal hypertension including splenomegaly and ascites may be present. Jaundice is present in approximately half of patients.

Diagnostic Evaluation

Laboratory examination may reveal abnormal liver function tests. Alpha-fetoprotein is a specific marker for hepatoma but can also be elevated in embryonic tumors. Radiographic studies are used to differentiate benign and malignant lesions. Ultrasonography can distinguish cystic from solid lesions, whereas CT or magnetic resonance imaging can reveal multiple lesions and clarify anatomic relationships. Hepatic arteriography can diagnose a hemangioma.

Treatment

Treatment involves resection of the tumor. Survival without treatment averages 3 months; resection can extend survival to 3 years, with a 5-year survival of 11–46%. The decision to resect the tumor depends on comorbid disease and the location and size of the tumor. When possible, wedge resection should be performed as formal hepatic lobectomy does not improve survival.

Metastatic disease occurs in decreasing frequency from bronchogenic, colon, pancreatic, breast, and stomach. When colon cancer metastasizes to the liver, resection of up to three lesions has been shown to improve survival and should be attempted as long as the operative risk is not prohibitive. In general, liver metastases from other tumors should not be resected.

Key Points

1. Hepatocellular carcinoma is extremely common worldwide but relatively rare in the United States.
2. Causes of hepatocellular carcinoma include cirrhosis, aflatoxin, smoking, and vinyl chloride.
3. Prognosis for hepatocellular carcinoma is poor.

▶ LIVER ABSCESSES

Etiology

Liver abscesses are most frequently due to bacteria, amebas, or the tapeworm echinococcus. Bacterial abscesses usually arise from an intra-abdominal infection in the appendix, gallbladder, or intestine but may be due to trauma, or a complication of a surgical procedure. Causative organisms are principally gut flora including *Escherichia coli, Klebsiella, Enterococcus,* and anaerobes including bacteroides. Amebic abscesses are an infrequent complication of gastrointestinal amebiasis.

Epidemiology

Pyogenic abscesses are responsible for less than 1 in 500 adult hospital admissions. Amebic abscesses occur in 3 to 25% of patients with gastrointestinal amebiasis. Risk factors include human immunodeficiency virus, alcohol abuse, and foreign travel. Echinococcus is most commonly seen in eastern Europe, Greece, South Africa, South America, and Australia; although rare in the United States, they are the most common cause of liver abscesses worldwide.

History

Patients with pyogenic or amebic abscess usually have nonspecific complaints of vague abdominal pain, weight loss, malaise, anorexia, and fever. Travel to an endemic region may suggest echinococcus.

Physical Examination

The liver may be tender or enlarged, and jaundice may occur. Rupture of an abscess can lead to peritonitis, sepsis, and circulatory collapse.

Diagnostic Evaluation

The white blood cell count and transaminase levels are elevated. Antibodies to ameba are found in 98% of patients with amebic abscesses but less than 5% of patients with pyogenic abscesses. Echinococcal infection produces eosinophilia and a positive heme agglutination test. Ultrasonography is approximately 90% sensitive for demonstrating a lesion, and CT is slightly better. The presence of multiple cysts or "sand" on CT is suggestive of echinococcus. Sampling of the cyst contents with CT or ultrasound guidance will reveal the causative organism in the case of pyogenic abscesses but will not usually lead to a diagnosis in amebic abscesses. Aspiration of echinococcal cysts is contraindicated because of the risk of contamination of the peritoneal cavity.

Treatment

Pyogenic abscesses require antibiotics alone or in combination with percutaneous or open drainage. Amebic abscesses are treated with flagyl with or without chloroquine, and surgical drainage is reserved for complications including rupture. Echinococcal abscess requires an open procedure. Scolicidal agents (e.g., ethanol or 20% sodium chloride) are instilled directly into the cyst. This is followed by drainage, with care not to spill the organisms into the peritoneum.

Key Point

Liver abscesses

1. Are most commonly caused by bacteria, amebas, or echinococcus.

▶ PORTAL HYPERTENSION

Etiology

Portal hypertension is caused by processes that impede hepatic blood flow either at the presinusoidal, sinusoidal, or postsinusoidal levels. Presinusoidal causes include schistosomiasis and portal vein thrombosis. The principal sinusoidal cause in the United States is cirrhosis, most commonly caused by alcohol, but also by hepatitis B and C. Approximately 15% of alcoholics will develop cirrhosis. Postsinusoidal causes of portal hypertension include Budd-Chiari syndrome (hepatic vein occlusion), pericarditis, and right-sided heart failure.

Complications

Bleeding varices are a life-threatening complication of portal hypertension. When portal pressures rise, collateralization through the hemorrhoidal, umbilical, or coronary veins becomes the low resistance route for blood flow. The coronary vein empties into the plexus of veins draining the stomach and esophagus (Fig. 10-2).Engorgement of these veins places the patient at risk of bleeding into the esophagus or stomach.

History

Alcoholism, hepatitis, or previous variceal hemorrhages are common.

Physical Examination

A variety of physical findings including ascites, jaundice, cherubic face, spider angiomata, testicular atrophy, gynecomastia, and palmar erythema may suggest the diagnosis.

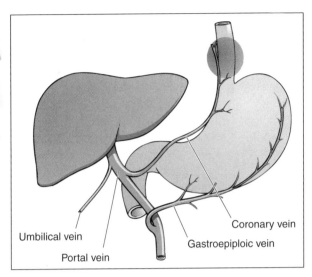

Figure 10-2 Selected collateral circulation in portal hypertension.

Diagnostic Evaluation

Laboratory examination may reveal increased liver enzymes, but these may return to normal with advanced cirrhosis as the amount of functioning hepatic parenchyma decreases. For unknown reasons, an alanine aminotransferase (ALT) to aspartate aminotransferase (AST) ratio of greater than 2 suggests alcohol as the etiology for cirrhosis. Tests of liver synthetic function may be abnormal, including clotting times and serum albumin.

Treatment

For patients with upper gastrointestinal bleeds, large-bore intravenous lines and volume resuscitation should be started immediately. A nasogastric tube should be placed to confirm the diagnosis. If the patient cannot be lavaged clear, suggesting active bleeding, emergent endoscopy is both diagnostic and therapeutic. Endoscopy is greater than 90% effective in controlling acute bleeding from esophageal varices. Should this fail, balloon tamponade or vasopressin infusion should be considered. Should these methods fail, a surgical shunting procedure should be considered.

The incidence of variceal bleed in a patient with varices is 30–50%, but this increases to 70% in someone with a previous variceal bleed. For this reason, a definitive procedure should be considered after the initial episode is controlled.

Key Points

1. Portal hypertension has presinusoidal, sinusoidal, and postsinusoidal causes.

2. Variceal hemorrhage is life-threatening, but endoscopy is usually successful in controlling bleeding.

3. Because of the high recurrence rate, a definitive procedure should be considered after the first episode of variceal bleeding.

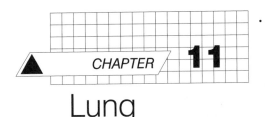

CHAPTER 11

Lung

▶ ANATOMY

The lung is divided into three lobes and 10 segments on the right and two lobes and nine segments on the left. The decreased number of divisions on the left can be thought of as space taken up by the heart. The right mainstem bronchus forms a more gentle curve into the trachea than does the left mainstem bronchus, and aspiration of foreign bodies or gastric contents is more likely to affect the right lung (Fig. 11-1), specifically the dependent portions that are the superior segment of the right lower lobe and the posterior segment of the right upper lobe. Arterial supply to the lung is through the pulmonary artery as well as the bronchial arteries, which arise from the aorta and intercostal vessels.

▶ BENIGN TUMORS OF THE TRACHEA AND BRONCHI

Pathology

Types include squamous papillomatosis, angioma, fibroma, leiomyoma, and chondroma. Squamous papillomatosis is associated with human papilloma viruses 6 and 11.

Epidemiology

Truly benign neoplasms of the trachea and bronchi are rare.

History

Patients commonly present with recurrent pneumonias, cough, or hemoptysis.

Physical Examination

Patients may have decreased breath sounds.

Diagnostic Evaluation

Chest radiograph may demonstrate a mass, and there may be a postobstructive pneumonia if the lesion narrows the bronchial lumen.

Treatment

Angiomas frequently regress, and observation is recommended. Surgical removal is necessary for the other lesions to relieve symptoms and establish a diagnosis. This frequently requires reanastomosis of a bronchus or the trachea. Squamous papillomatosis has a high recurrence rate.

Key Point

1. Benign lesions of the trachea and bronchi are rare.

▶ TUMORS WITH MALIGNANT POTENTIAL

The group includes bronchial carcinoids, adenoid cystic carcinoma, and mucoepidermoid tumors. They do not usually show invasive or metastatic features, but a subset of each of these tumors does. Carcinoid tumors are malignant in approximately 10% of patients. They are known for their ability to release a variety of substances including histamine, serotonin, vasoactive intestinal peptide, gastrin, growth hormone, insulin, glucagon, and catecholamines.

Epidemiology

These tumors comprise less than 5% of all pulmonary neoplasms and have no obvious age or sex predilection. Carcinoids comprise approximately 1% of all lung tumors, adenoid cystic carcinoma approximately 0.5%, and mucoepidermoid approximately 0.2%.

History

Patients most commonly complain of cough, dyspnea, hemoptysis, or recurrent pneumonia. Carcinoid tumors may produce carcinoid syndrome, and the patient may complain of flushing and diarrhea, as well as manifestations of specific hormone excess. This syndrome occurs in approximately 3% of patients with carcinoid tumors.

Physical Examination

Patient may have respiratory compromise or decreased breath sounds. Carcinoid tumors may cause valvular heart disease with signs of pulmonic stenosis and tricuspid regurgitation.

Diagnostic Evaluation

Chest radiograph may reveal a lesion or pneumonia. Bronchoscopy is useful to obtain tissue diagnosis. Computed tomography (CT) or magnetic resonance imaging will identify the site of the lesion to plan surgical treatment.

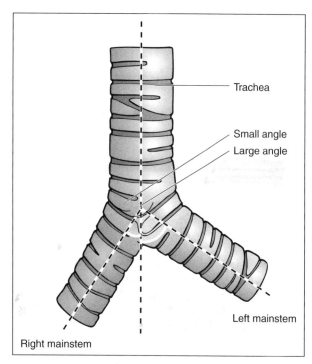

Figure 11-1 Anatomy of the mainstem bronchi.

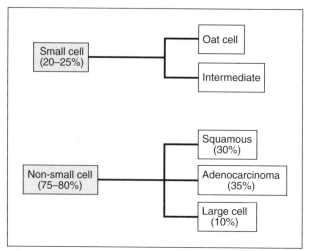

Figure 11-2 Division of lung cancer.

Treatment

These tumors should all be resected. Long-term survival for carcinoid tumors is 80%; for adenoid cystic carcinoma and mucoepidermoid tumors the prognosis is also favorable.

Key Point

Carcinoid tumors

1. Can release a variety of substances causing paraneoplastic syndromes.

▶ LUNG CANCER

Epidemiology

Malignant lesions of the lung are the most common malignancies in both men and women. They are responsible for approximately 150,000 deaths each year. Smoking is responsible in approximately 80% of cases, but exposure to formaldehyde, radon gas, asbestos, arsenic, uranium, chromates, and nickel have also been identified as etiologic agents.

Pathology

Lung cancer is divided into small cell (20–25%) and non-small cell carcinoma (75–80%). Small cell carcinoma is further divided into oat cell and intermediate cell types. Non-small cell is further divided into squamous cell carcinoma (30%), adenocarcinoma (35%),

and large cell carcinoma (10%) (Fig. 11-2). Small cell cancer is usually central, and this form of cancer may be associated with paraneoplastic syndromes. Approximately 5% will have symptoms of inappropriate secretion of antidiuretic hormone, whereas 3–5% will have Cushing's syndrome from ACTH production. Squamous cell cancer usually occurs centrally and can be associated with symptoms of hypercalcemia secondary to production of a substance similar to parathyroid hormone. Adenocarcinoma typically occurs at the periphery.

History

Patients commonly complain of hemoptysis or obstructive symptoms of cough, dyspnea, and pneumonia. Systemic symptoms including weight loss are common. Symptoms of advanced disease include chest pain from local invasion. Bone pain may signify metastatic disease.

Physical Examination

Changes in voice due to invasion of the recurrent laryngeal nerve and Horner's syndrome (ptosis, myosis, and anhydrosis) may result from a tumor in the superior sulcus causing neural compression. Superior vena cava syndrome and Pancoast's syndrome (shoulder and arm pain on the affected side) may occur. The phrenic nerve may be involved resulting in paralysis of the hemidiaphragm. Neurologic deficits, jaundice or hepatomegaly, and pathologic fractures may be due to metastases to brain, liver, or bone.

Diagnostic Evaluation

Although screening chest radiograph has not been shown to improve survival, it is often the modality for first discovery of the lesion. Chest CT will delineate the size and location of the lesion for help with staging. Because of the propensity for metastases, bone scan, head CT, and liver function tests should be obtained. Bronchoscopic tissue biopsy and cells obtained from bronchial washing will help establish the diagnosis. Mediastinoscopy with lymph node biopsy will allow accurate staging and possibly tissue diagnosis (for staging, see Table 11-1).

TABLE 11-1

Current International Staging System for Non-Small Cell Lung Cancer

Staging

Primary tumor (T)

TX   Tumor proved by the presence of malignant cells in bronchopulmonary secretions but not visualized roentgenographically or bronchoscopically, or any tumor that cannot be assessed as in a retreatment staging

TO   No evidence of primary tumor

Tis   Carcinoma in situ

T1*   A tumor that is 3 cm or less in greatest dimension, surrounded by lung or visceral pleura, and without evidence of invasion proximal to a lobar bronchus at bronchoscopy

T2   A tumor more than 3 cm in greatest dimension, or a tumor of any size that either invades the visceral pleura or has associated atelectasis or obstructive pneumonitis extending to the hilar region. At bronchoscopy, the proximal extent of demonstrable tumor must be within a lobar bronchus or at least 2 cm distal to the carina. Any associated atelectasis or obstructive pneumonitis must involve less than an entire lung

T3   A tumor of any size with direct extension into the chest wall (including superior sulcus tumors), diaphragm, or the mediastinal pleura or pericardium without involving the heart, great vessels, trachea, esophagus, or vertebral body, or a tumor in the main bronchus within 2 cm of the carina without involving the carina

T4†   A tumor of any size with invasion of the mediastinum or involving the heart, great vessels, trachea, esophagus, vertebral body, or carina or presence of malignant pleural effusion

Nodal involvement (N)

NO   No demonstrable metastasis to regional lymph nodes

N1   Metastasis to lymph nodes in the peribronchial or the ipsilateral hilar region, or both, including direct extension

N2   Metastasis to ipsilateral mediastinal lymph nodes and subcarinal lymph nodes

N3   Metastasis to contralateral mediastinal lymph nodes, contralateral hilar lymph nodes, ipsilateral or contralateral scalene lymph nodes, or supraclavicular lymph nodes

Distant metastasis (M)

MO   No (known) distant metastasis

M1   Distant metastasis present—specify sites

Stage grouping

Occult carcinoma	TX, NO, MO
Stage 0	Tis, carcinoma in situ
Stage I	T1, NO, MO
	T2, NO, MO
Stage II	T1, N1, MO
	T2, N1, MO
Stage IIIa	T3, NO, MO
	T3, N1, MO
	T1–3, N2, MO
Stage IIIb	Any T, N3, MO
	T4, any N, MO
Stage IV	Any T, any N, M1

*The uncommon superficial tumor of any size with its invasive component limited to the bronchial wall that may extend proximal to the main bronchus is classified as T1.

†Most pleural effusions associated with lung cancer are due to tumor. There are, however, some few patients in whom cytopathologic examination of pleural fluid (on more than one specimen) is negative for tumor and in whom the fluid is nonbloody and is not an exudate. In cases in which these elements and clinical judgment dictate that the effusion is not related to the tumor, the patient should be staged T1, T2, or T3, excluding effusion as a staging element.

Treatment

Resection of small cell lung cancer is indicated only if the lesion is well localized, which is rare. The disease is usually widely disseminated at the time of diagnosis, and chemotherapy is the mainstay of treatment. Common regimens include doxorubicin, cyclophosphamide, and vincristine. Radiation therapy, especially prophylactically to the brain, should be considered.

Treatment of non-small cell lung cancer includes surgery for stage I and II lesions, as well as certain stage III lesions. Radiation should be considered for locally advanced lesions; the usefulness of chemotherapy for these lesions is unclear.

Prognosis

Only approximately 50% of patients have resectable disease at presentation, and 5-year survival for all patients is just over 10%. For resectable non-small cell stage I lesions, the 5-year survival is 80%, but this figure drops to 30% for resectable stage II disease. Long-term survival in small cell cancer is rare.

Key Points

Lung cancer

1. Is the most common cause of cancer death in both men and women;

2. Surgical treatment is usually limited to non-small cell cancer, but prognosis is poor.

▶ MESOTHELIOMA

Pathology

This is a malignant lesion derived most commonly from the visceral pleura.

Epidemiology

The tumor is rare. Asbestos is the major risk factor. Cigarette smoking markedly increases the incidence of mesothelioma in patients exposed to asbestos.

History

Chest pain from local extension, dyspnea, and fever may occur.

Physical Examination

The patient may have decreased breath sounds on the side of the tumor due to a pleural effusion.

Diagnostic Evaluation

Chest radiograph will often demonstrate a pleural effusion. Thoracocentesis typically yields bloody fluid. Cytology may identify malignant cells. Patients with a suggestive history and a pleural effusion with no other explanation should undergo pleuroscopy and pleural biopsy even in the presence of negative fluid cytology.

Treatment

Survival beyond 2 years is rare. Extrapleural pneumonectomy that involves removal of the entire pleura and lung on the affected side may provide long-term survival. Chemotherapy and radiation therapy are experimental modalities at this time.

Key Points

1. Asbestos is the major risk factor for mesothelioma. Cigarette smoking greatly increases the risk.

2. Prognosis for mesothelioma is poor.

▶ PNEUMOTHORAX

The lung is covered by visceral pleura, and the inner chest wall is covered by parietal pleura. These two surfaces form a potential space. Simple pneumothorax occurs when air enters this space. Open pneumothorax occurs when a defect in the chest wall allows continuous entry of air from the outside. Tension pneumothorax occurs when a defect in the visceral pleura allows air to enter the potential space but not to escape. A valve-like effect allows pressure to increase and forcibly collapse the ipsilateral lung and mediastinal structures.

Etiology

Spontaneous pneumothorax most commonly occurs in young thin males or in those with bullous emphysema. It can also occur in patients on mechanical ventilation, especially if high inspiratory pressures are required. Infection, specifically tuberculosis or *Pneumocystis carinii*, can cause pneumothorax, as can lung tumors. Placement of central venous catheters results in pneumothorax in 1% of cases. Thoracocentesis, needle biopsy, or operative trauma are other iatrogenic causes. Open pneumothorax is caused by trauma, whereas tension pneumothorax can occur by any of the above mechanisms.

History

Patients can be asymptomatic or complain of sudden or gradual onset of dyspnea and pleuritic chest pain.

Physical Examination

Simple pneumothorax may result in decreased breath sounds and hyper-resonance on the affected side. Tension pneumothorax may cause decreased venous return and shock, and the trachea may be displaced away from the affected side.

Diagnostic Evaluation

Chest radiograph will reveal absence of lung markings in the affected area, usually in the apex in an upright film. Tracheal deviation or mediastinal shift suggests tension pneumothorax.

Treatment

Simple pneumothoracies of less than 20% can be observed with a trial of supplemental oxygen. Indications for tube thoracostomy include larger lesions or those which increase in size. Open pneumothorax requires repair of the defect and tube thoracostomy. Tension pneumothorax is a surgical emergency and requires needle thoracostomy, usually in the midclavicular line in the second intercostal space on the affected side. This should decompress the chest and allow blood return to the heart. Tube thoracostomy should follow on an emergent basis.

Key Point

Tension pneumothorax

1. Is a surgical emergency.

▶ EMPYEMA

Empyema is an infected pleural effusion.

Etiology

They are most commonly caused by pneumonia, lung abscess, prior thoracic surgery, or esophageal perforation. The most common organisms are ones causing primary lung infection, including staph, strep, pseudomonas, *Klebsiella, Escherichia coli*, proteus, and bacteroides.

History

There may be history of previous pneumonia, thoracic surgery, or esophageal instrumentation. Fatigue, lethargy, and shaking chills may occur.

Physical Examination

The patient may appear systemically sick. Fever and decreased breath sounds at the affected lung base are common.

Diagnostic Evaluation

The white blood cell count is elevated. Chest radiograph may reveal an effusion. Aspiration of the fluid will show a transudate characterized by pH less than 7.2 and high LDH. White blood cells and bacteria on Gram stain and culture may be present.

Treatment

Occasionally, antibiotics and needle aspiration alone are successful, but usually tube thoracostomy is required.

Key Point

Empyema

1. Is usually treated with tube thoracostomy and antibiotics.

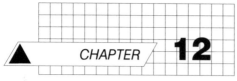

CHAPTER 12

Male Genitourinary System

▶ BENIGN PROSTATIC HYPERPLASIA

Benign prostatic hyperplasia (BPH) is a common benign condition of the prostate gland seen in older men. BPH is clinically important because it is the most common cause of bladder outlet obstruction in men over 50 years of age. If left untreated, bladder outlet obstruction can lead to urinary tract infection and bladder stones secondary to stasis from incomplete bladder emptying, bladder decompensation resulting in chronic urinary retention with overflow, and, most serious of all, renal failure secondary to high pressure urinary retention.

Pathogenesis

Prostate gland growth is influenced by steroid hormones. However, the exact mechanism of prostatic hyperplasia remains unclear. Interestingly, BPH does not occur in castrated men or pseudohermaphrodites, both of which lack the active metabolite of testosterone, dihydrotestosterone (DHT). Estrogens have also been implicated in prostatic hyperplasia, because in aging men, the levels of estrogens rise and those of androgens fall.

The specific area of cellular hyperplasia is the transitional zone or periurethral area of the prostate. The periurethral glandular elements undergo hyperplasia, causing an increase in glandular mass that results in compression of the prostatic urethra and the onset of obstructive symptoms (Fig. 12-1).

Epidemiology

The prevalence of BPH increases with age. Autopsy studies show that at least 50% of men over the age of 50 have significant enlargement of the prostate due to BPH. Rarely does a patient present before the age of 50, because the doubling time of the hyperplastic gland is slow. By age 90, roughly 90% of males will have a significant degree of hyperplasia. All men with intact functional testis are at risk for developing BPH.

Clinical Manifestations

History

Any older man presenting with obstructive urinary symptoms must be suspected of having BPH. Symptoms include hesitancy, poor stream, a sensation of incomplete bladder emptying after voiding, nocturia, or terminal dribbling. Occasionally, an elderly male patient will present with hematuria after straining at urination. The pressure from straining has caused rupture of an engorged mucosal vessel covering the hyperplastic gland. Secondary symptoms are a consequence of urinary stasis. High postvoid residual volumes promote bacterial growth, leading to urinary tract infection. Stasis can also promote the formation of bladder calculi. Most seriously, high pressure chronic retention can cause bilateral hydroureteronephrosis and subsequent renal failure.

Physical Examination

A careful rectal examination reveals an enlarged symmetric rubbery gland. The size of the gland has no relationship to symptomatology. A small gland may produce a high degree of outflow obstruction, whereas a large gland may produce no symptoms at all. Posterior enlargement with compression of the anterior rectal wall can occasionally produce constipation. The suprapubic region should be palpated to rule out a grossly distended bladder.

Diagnostic Evaluation

Urine should be obtained for sediment analysis and microbiologic cultures. Serum blood urea nitrogen and creatinine levels should be checked for evidence of renal insufficiency. If chronic urinary retention is suspected, a postvoid residual may be checked by straight catheterization. Urinary flow rate is assessed by measuring the volume of urine voided during a 5-second period. A flow rate of less than 50 mL in 5 seconds is evidence of bladder outlet obstruction. Ultrasonography is the preferred modality for imaging the urinary tract. Information regarding size of the prostate, presence of bladder stones, the postvoid residual volume, and hydronephrosis can be obtained. Transabdominal ultrasound has replaced the once routine intravenous pyelogram while transrectal ultrasonography is used to evaluate an irregular prostate when found on examination or an elevated prostate-specific antigen (PSA) level.

Treatment

The goals of drug therapy for BPH are to relax smooth muscle in the prostate and bladder neck and to induce

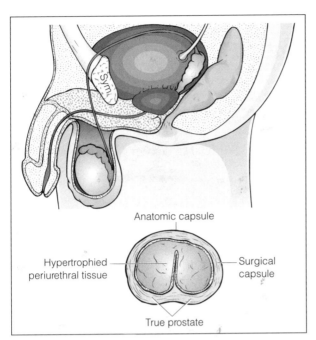

Figure 12-1 Benign prostatic hyperplasia causing urethral compression. The enlarged periurethral glands are enclosed by the orange-peel like surgical capsule which is composed of compressed true prostatic tissue.

regression of cellular hyperplasia, thereby enhancing urinary outflow from the bladder to the urethra. Alpha-blockade of adrenergic receptors produces smooth muscle relaxation of both prostate and bladder neck. A common side-effect of alpha-antagonists (e.g., terazosin) is postural hypotension. Prostatic hyperplasia is treated with 5-alpha-reductase inhibitors (e.g., finasteride) that block the conversion of testosterone to DHT without lowering serum levels of circulation testosterone.

Surgical relief of obstruction is necessary when medical therapy fails. The indications for surgery are a postvoid residual volume greater than 100 mL, acute urinary retention, chronic urinary retention with overflow dribbling, gross hematuria on more than one occasion, and recurrent urinary tract infections. Additional indications are patient request for restoration of normal urodynamics because of excessive nocturia or dribbling.

The procedure of choice is transurethral resection of the prostate (TURP). With the patient in the lithotomy position, the resectoscope is introduced via the urethra into the bladder. The occlusive prostate tissue is identified, and under direct vision, the tissue is shaved away using an electrified wire loop. As the bladder is constantly irrigated with a nonelectrolytic isotonic solution, extravasated blood and tissue fragments are evacuated. An indwelling catheter is left in place for 3 to 4 days.

Key Points

Benign prostatic hyperplasia

1. Is a disease of older men that causes bladder outlet obstruction;
2. Obstructive urinary symptoms include hesitancy, poor stream, incomplete bladder emptying, nocturia, and dribbling;
3. Secondary symptoms arising from urinary stasis include urinary tract infections, bladder calculi, hydroureteronephrosis, and renal failure;
4. Is medically treated by alpha-blockade to relax prostate and bladder neck smooth muscle and 5-alpha-reductase inhibition to block DHT production and cause regression of cellular hyperplasia;
5. Is surgically treated by TURP.

▶ TESTES

Disorders of the testes requiring surgical management include congenital abnormalities, tumors, and, in the emergent setting, testicular torsion.

Congenital Abnormalities
Cryptorchidism

This is the failure of normal testicular descent during embryologic development. The cause of failed descent is unknown but may be due to a selective hormone deficiency. Such cryptorchid testes fail in spermatogenic function, but they may retain ability to secrete androgens.

Physical Examination   The testicle remains within the abdomen and is unable to be palpated on physical examination.

Treatment   Because spermatogenic failure is progressive, surgical exploration and scrotal placement of the testis should be performed before 2 years of age. If placement of the testicle into the scrotum is not possible, then orchiectomy is indicated because the incidence of cancer of abdominal testes is very high. Because diagnosis is usually not made before age 10, orchiectomy is the usual treatment because of cancer risk and poor spermatogenesis.

Incomplete Descent of the Testis

This implies a testicle arrested at some point in the path of normal descent but palpable on physical examination. Such testes are usually located within the inguinal canal between the deep and superficial rings. Incompletely descended testes are often associated with congenital indirect hernias due to the incomplete obliteration of the process vaginalis.

Treatment Because testicular function is less compromised than a cryptorchid testis, the usual treatment is repositioning and orchiopexy within the scrotum. If present, the indirect hernia is repaired concurrently.

Testicular Tumors

Tumors of the testicle are the most common genitourinary malignancy among young men between the ages of 20 and 35 years. Virtually all neoplasms of the testicle are malignant. Tumors are divided into either germ cell or non-germ cell tumors, depending on their cellular origin. Germ cell tumors predominate, accounting for 90% to 95% of all tumors.

Pathology

Non-germ cell tumors arise from Leydig and Sertoli cells and produce excess quantities of androgenizing hormones. Germ cell tumors arise from totipotential cells of the seminiferous tubules. There are several germ cell tumor types, categorized according to the degree of cellular differentiation: seminoma, embryonal carcinoma, and choriocarcinoma. Seminomas are relatively slow growing and exhibit late invasion. They are usually discovered and surgically removed before metastasis can occur. Embryonal carcinomas are less differentiated than seminomas and exhibit greater malignant behavior and metastasize earlier. Choriocarcinomas are highly invasive aggressive tumors that metastasize via lymphatic and venous systems early in the disease course.

Epidemiology

Seminomas are the most common malignant germ cell tumor. Embryonal carcinoma is usually seen in younger males during childhood. Non-germ cell tumors are relatively rare.

History

Tumors usually present as firm painless testicular masses. Occasionally, the mass may cause a dull ache. Hemorrhage into necrotic tumor or after minor trauma may cause the acute onset of pain. About 10% of patients with testicular tumors have a history of cryptorchidism. Because of excess androgen production, non-germ cell tumors can cause precocious puberty and virilism in young males and impotence and gynecomastia in adults.

Diagnostic Evaluation

Immediate evaluation should include serum for tumor markers (alpha-fetoprotein [AFP], beta-human chorionic gonadotropin [β-hCG]) and tissue biopsy for definitive diagnosis. Tumor markers are not always helpful because seminomas, the most common testicular neoplasm, usually are negative for both AFP and β-hCG. In neoplasms with tumor markers, the level of tumor burden directly relates to AFP/β-hCG levels that can be followed during the postoperative period to evaluate the efficacy of treatment and to detect recurrence.

Treatment

Treatment decisions are based on tumor histology and staging of disease. Surgical intervention usually involves orchiectomy ± retroperitoneal lymph node dissection. For bulky tumors, surgery may follow chemotherapy to evaluate for residual disease. If residual malignancy is found, then chemotherapy is continued.

Seminomas are usually highly radiosensitive. Adjuvant treatment with radiation and chemotherapy yields high 5-year survival rates for both localized and metastatic disease. Embryonal carcinoma exhibits high malignant potential and early metastasis. Choriocarcinoma is usually widely metastatic at diagnosis. Prognosis is poor for both tumor types despite chemotherapy.

Torsion of the Testicle

Testicular torsion is a urologic emergency because complete strangulation of the blood supply renders the testicle surgically unsalvageable after about 6 hours.

Pathogenesis

Torsion results from an abnormally high attachment of the tunica vaginalis around the distal end of the spermatic cord, which allows the testis to hang within the tunica compartment like a bell clapper within a bell, hence the name, bell clapper deformity, in which the testicle is free to twist on its own blood supply, causing pain and ischemic strangulation (Fig. 12-2).

History

Torsion is usually seen in young males who present complaining of the rapid onset of severe testicle pain, followed by testicle swelling.

Physical examination reveals a high riding, swollen, tender testicle, oriented horizontally in the scrotum.

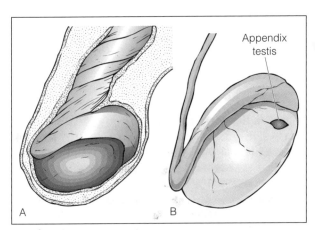

Figure 12-2 Torsion of the testes (A) is the result of twisting of the spermatic cord, usually within the tunica vaginalis; the appendix testis may also become twisted (B).

Diagnostic Evaluation

A color-flow Doppler ultrasound should be obtained to evaluate for blood flow within the testicle. Absence of flow confirms the diagnosis.

Differential Diagnosis

The differential diagnosis of an acutely swollen tender testicle includes essentially two diagnoses: torsion of the spermatic cord and advanced epididymitis. As one can mimic the other, it is vitally important to arrive at a timely diagnosis. Other lesser diagnoses include torsion of an appendix testis or appendix epididymis.

Treatment

Once the diagnosis is confirmed, prompt surgical exploration and orchiopexy is required to save the testicle.

Because the bell clapper deformity is usually bilateral, orchiopexy of the contralateral testicle is performed concurrently. If the diagnosis is unclear, surgical exploration is required because an uncorrected torsion has catastrophic consequences.

Key Points

Cryptorchidism and incomplete testicular descent

1. Are congenital abnormalities;
2. Abdominal testes have a high incidence of cancer.

Testicular tumors

1. Are either germ cell tumors (seminomas [the most common], embryonal carcinoma, choriocarcinoma) or non-germ cell tumors (Leydig and Sertoli cell tumors);
2. Usually present as firm painless testicular masses;
3. AFP and β-hCG measurement and tissue biopsy are used for diagnosis;
4. Orchiectomy is standard treatment ± radiation.

Testicular torsion

1. Is caused by abnormally high attachment of the tunical vaginalis around the distal end of the spermatic cord;
2. Is evaluated by Doppler ultrasound because epididymitis can mimic torsion;
3. Requires prompt surgical exploration and bilateral orchiopexy to reverse the ischemic strangulation of torsion.

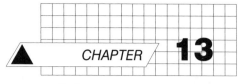

CHAPTER 13

Neurosurgery

▶ BRAIN TUMORS

Because the brain is encased in a nonexpandable bony skull, both benign and malignant brain tumors can cause death if not appropriately diagnosed and treated. Most brain tumors eventually cause elevated intracranial pressure (ICP), either by occupying space, producing cerebral edema, interfering with the normal flow of cerebrospinal fluid, or impairing venous drainage. At presentation, patients usually complain of progressive neurologic deficits and worsening symptoms attributable to rising ICP, tumor invasion, and brain compression (Fig. 13-1).

Pathology

Intracranial tumors can be classified as either intracerebral or extracerebral tumors (Table 13-1). Intracerebral tumors include glial cell tumors (astrocytomas, oligodendrogliomas, ependymomas, medulloblastomas), metastatic tumors (lung, breast, melanoma, kidney, colon), pineal gland tumors, and papillomas of the choroid plexus. Extracerebral tumors arise from extracerebral structures and include meningiomas, acoustic neuromas, pituitary adenomas, and craniopharyngiomas.

Glial cell tumors and metastatic tumors are the most common central nervous system (CNS) tumors seen in adults, whereas tumors of the posterior fossa are most commonly seen in children.

Glial Cell Tumors

Tumors of glial cells account for approximately 50% of CNS tumors seen in adults. Different glial cell types (astrocytes, oligodendrocytes, ependymal cells, and neuroglial precursors) give rise to various histologic types of tumors. Although the term "glioma" can be used to describe the above glial tumor types, its common use refers only to astrocytic tumors.

Astrocytic tumors are graded according to histologic evidence of malignancy using a three-point scale. Slow-growing astrocytomas are the least malignant and are designated grade I tumors. In children, astrocytomas located in the posterior fossa (cerebellum) usually have cystic morphologies. The more aggressive anaplastic astrocytomas are grade II. The most common and also the most malignant astrocytoma is the grade III glioblastoma multiforme (GBM). GBM tumors often track through the white matter, crossing the midline via the corpus callosum, resulting in the so-called "butterfly glioma" on CT. Survival with GBM lesions is less than 1 year.

Oligodendrogliomas are slow-growing tumors often seen in the frontal lobes. They are mostly seen in adults and often have evidence of calcifications on plain radiographs.

Ependymomas arise from cells that line the ventricular walls and central canal. Clinical signs and symptoms of elevated ICP are the main features of presentation. Ependymomas are mostly seen in children and usually arise in the fourth ventricle.

Infratentorial posterior fossa tumors comprise most of the lesions seen in childhood. Cystic cerebellar astrocytomas, ependymomas, and medulloblastomas account for most of these tumors. Highly malignant medulloblastomas are essentially cerebellar tumors, seen in the vermis in children and in the cerebellar hemispheres in young adults.

Metastatic Tumors

About 30% of patients with systemic cancer will have cerebral metastases, which usually originate in the lung, breast, skin (melanoma), kidney, and colon. Most lesions are supratentorial, located in the distribution of the middle meningeal artery. Single approachable lesions can be surgically removed, but radiotherapy is the usual treatment.

Meningiomas

Slow-growing meningiomas arise from the lining of the brain and spinal cord. Complete tumor removal is curative and residual disease responds to radiotherapy.

History

Patients usually present with neurologic signs and symptoms attributable to cerebral compression from the expanding tumor mass. Headache, nausea, and vomiting are the most common generalized symptoms of elevated ICP. Classically, patients complain of diffuse headache that is worse in the morning after a night of recumbency.

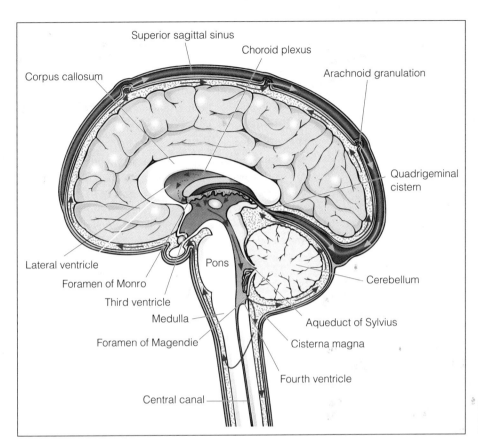

Superior sagittal sinus
Choroid plexus
Corpus callosum
Arachnoid granulation
Quadrigeminal cistern
Lateral ventricle
Pons
Cerebellum
Foramen of Monro
Third ventricle
Medulla
Aqueduct of Sylvius
Foramen of Magendie
Cisterna magna
Fourth ventricle
Central canal

Figure 13-1 Pathways for the circulation of cerebrospinal fluid.

TABLE 13-1

Intracranial Tumors

Intracerebral
  Glial cell tumors—astrocytomas, anaplastic astrocytomas, glioblastoma multiforme, oligodendroglioma, ependymoma, medulloblastoma
  Metastatic tumors—lung, breast, melanoma, kidney, colon
  Pineal gland tumors
  Papillomas of the choroid plexus
Extracerebral
  Meningiomas
  Neuromas, especially acoustic neuromas
  Pituitary tumors
  Craniopharyngiomas
  Hemangioblastomas of the cerebellum

Physical Examination

Bilateral papilledema is often present. Personality changes may be noted early on, which progress to stupor and coma as the ICP increases and brain herniation occurs (Fig. 13-2). Generalized seizures occasionally occur in tumors affecting the sensorimotor cortex.

Focal signs and symptoms occur when local areas of brain become functionally impaired. Focal sensory and motor loss are most common.

DDx

Intracerebral hemorrhage, neurodegenerative diseases, abscess, vascular malformations, meningitis, encephalitis, congenital hydrocephalus, toxic state.

Diagnostic Evaluation

CT and MRI assist in making the diagnosis and in localization of the tumor. MRI with gadolinium enhancement is useful for visualizing low-grade gliomas.

Treatment

Correct management of brain tumors requires knowledge of the natural history of specific tumor types and the risks associated with surgical removal. When feasible, total tumor removal is the goal; however, subtotal resection may be necessary if vital brain function is threatened by complete tumor extirpation. If subtotal resection is performed, postoperative radiation therapy can afford prolongation of life and palliation of symptoms. Chemotherapy is also used for specific tumor types.

Metastatic brain tumors are treated with whole-brain irradiation because most lesions are multiple. Occasionally, single lesions amenable to surgery are removed, followed by whole-brain irradiation.

Perioperative management of increased ICP due to cerebral edema is accomplished by using corticosteroids. If hydrocephalus is present, shunting may be required.

Key Points

1. Brain tumors cause elevated ICP by occupying space, producing cerebral edema, blocking cerebrospinal fluid flow, and impairing cerebral venous drainage, resulting in neurologic deficits.

2. Intracranial tumors are either intracerebral (glial cell tumors, metastatic tumors, pineal gland tumors, choroid plexus papillomas) or extracerebral (meningiomas, neuromas, pituitary tumors, hemangiomas).

3. GBM tumors are the most common and most malignant astrocytic tumors. They track across the corpus callosum and are called "butterfly gliomas."

4. Most childhood tumors are located in the posterior fossa and are cystic astrocytomas, ependymomas, and medulloblastomas.

Figure 13-2 Examples of brain herniation. 1, Cingulate gyrus herniation across the falx; 2, temporal uncus herniation across the tentorium; 3, cerebellar tonsil herniation through the foramen magnum; 4, herniation of brain tissue through craniotomy defect.

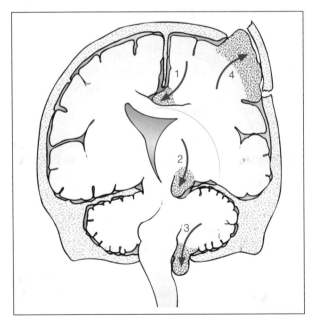

► INTRACRANIAL ANEURYSMS

Intracranial aneurysms are saccular "berry-shaped" aneurysms usually found at the arterial branch points within the circle of Willis (Fig. 13-3). Although they rarely rupture, significant morbidity and mortality may result secondary to hemorrhage. Subarachnoid hemorrhage develops when intracranial aneurysms bleed.

History

Sudden onset of a severe headache, typically described as the "worst headache of my life," usually signals the rupture of an intracranial aneurysm. ICP transiently rises with each cardiac contraction, causing a severe pulsating headache. Patients may develop progressive neurologic deficits due to mass effect, culminating in eventual coma and death.

A system for categorizing the severity of hemorrhage has been developed using clinical assessment based on neurologic condition. The five-point Hunt and Hess grading system ranges from grade I, indicating good neurologic condition, to grade 5, indicating significant neurologic deficits (Table 13-2).

Figure 13-3 Cerebral arterial circle of Willis.

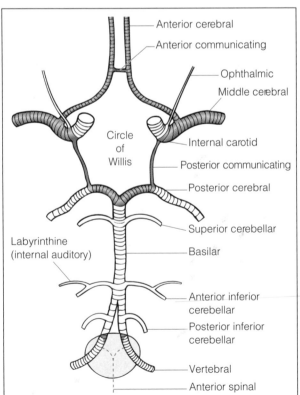

Diagnosis

CT is useful for demonstrating intracranial hemorrhage. For a more detailed study that defines the aneurysm neck and relationship with surrounding vessels, a four-vessel cerebral angiogram can be obtained (Fig. 13-4).

Treatment

Initial medical treatment involves tight control of hypertension with appropriate medications. Phenytoin is administered for prophylactic treatment of seizures, and mannitol may be given to control edema.

Neurosurgical intervention is indicated for high grade (4 to 5) disease with neurologic deficit. Emergent ventriculostomy is performed to lower the ICP. If the patient exhibits progressive neurologic deterioration, craniotomy is performed for removal of hematoma. The offending aneurysm is obliterated by microsurgical clipping of the sac.

Key Points

Intracranial aneurysms

1. Are usually found at arterial branch points within the circle of Willis;

2. Rupture causes severe headache and subarachnoid hemorrhage;

3. High-grade disease with neurologic deficit warrants neurosurgical intervention.

▶ EPIDURAL HEMATOMA

Epidural hematomas are usually seen in patients with head trauma who have sustained a skull fracture across the course of middle meningeal artery, causing an arterial laceration and an expanding hematoma (Fig. 13-5). The increasing pressure of the arterial-based hematoma strips the dura mater from the inner table of the skull, producing a lens-shaped mass capable of causing brain compression and herniation.

TABLE 13-2
Hunt-Hess Classification of Subarachnoid Hemorrhage

Grade	Description
1	Mild headache and slight nuchal rigidity
2	Cranial nerve palsy, severe headache, nuchal rigidity
3	Mild focal deficit, lethargy or confusion
4	Stupor, hemiparesis, early decerebrate rigidity
5	Deep coma, decerebrate rigidity, moribund appearance

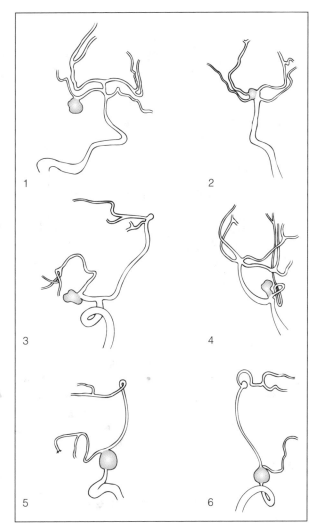

Figure 13-4 Drawings of six intracranial aneurysms as shown on vertebral angiograms.

History

Often the patient will have sustained head trauma without an initial neurologic deficit, who after a several hour "honeymoon" period experiences a rapidly progressive deterioration in their level of consciousness.

Physical Examination

The finding of a unilateral dilated pupil indicates brainstem herniation, whereas bilateral fixed and dilated pupils signal impending respiratory failure and death.

Diagnostic Evaluation

CT is crucial to establish a diagnosis and treatment plan.

Treatment

For patients presenting with a depressed skull fracture and a neurologic examination indicating a deteriorating

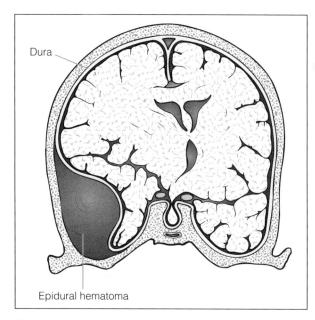

Figure 13-5 Epidural hemorrhage.

level of consciousness, emergent cranial decompression must be performed. A burr hole is made over the area of hematoma seen on CT, and the clot is decompressed with resultant lowering of the ICP. Once decompression is achieved, formal craniotomy can be performed to fully evacuate the clot and to control middle meningeal arterial bleeding.

Key Points

Epidural hematomas

1. Arise from middle meningeal artery hemorrhage after head trauma;

2. Produce a lens-shaped mass capable of causing brain herniation;

3. "Honeymoon" period may precede rapid progressive deterioration;

4. Emergent cranial decompression is lifesaving.

▶ SUBDURAL HEMATOMA

In contradistinction to epidural hematomas, subdural hematomas are low-pressure bleeds secondary to venous hemorrhage (Fig. 13-6). Both spontaneous and traumatic subdural bleeds occur. The source of hemorrhage is from ruptured bridging veins that drain blood from the brain into the superior sagittal sinus.

Risk Factors

Elderly patients with evidence of brain atrophy who take anticoagulation medications are at risk for developing subdural hematomas.

History

Headache and drowsiness are the usual presenting symptoms. Seizure activity and papilledema are uncommon. Patients with significant neurologic deficits secondary to mass effect may need urgent burr hole decompression or craniotomy.

Key Point

Subdural hematomas

1. Are low-pressure venous bleeds arising from ruptured bridging veins that drain blood from the brain into the superior sagittal sinus;

2. Elderly anticoagulated patients are at increased risk;

3. Neurologic deficit warrants neurosurgical intervention.

▶ SPINAL TUMORS

Tumors are defined by anatomic location as being either extradural, intradural, or intramedullary (Fig. 13-7). Extradural tumors are most commonly lesions of metastatic disease from primary cancers of the lung, breast, or prostate. Other common tumors are multiple myeloma of the spine and lymphoma. Back pain from cord compression is the usual presenting complaint.

Intradural tumors are located within the subarachnoid space. The most common tumors are meningiomas and neurofibromatomas. A nerve root tumor may transverse the intervertebral foramen into

Figure 13-6 Subdural hemorrhage.

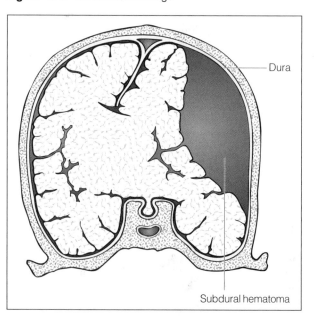

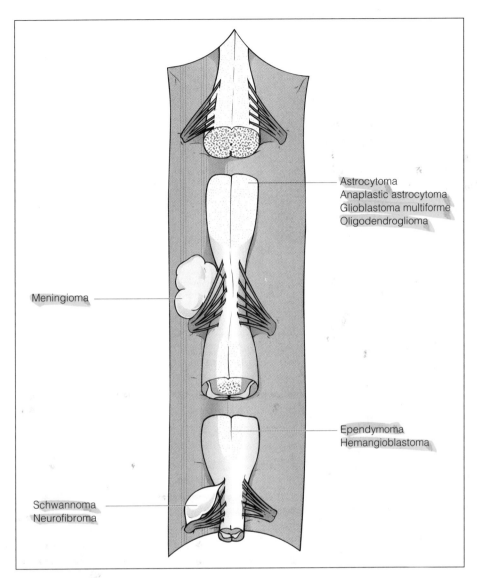

Astrocytoma
Anaplastic astrocytoma
Glioblastoma multiforme
Oligodendroglioma

Meningioma

Ependymoma
Hemangioblastoma

Schwannoma
Neurofibroma

Figure 13-7 Topographic distribution of the common neoplasms of the spinal meninges, spinal nerve roots, and spinal cord.

the extrathecal space, forming a bilobed lesion called a dumbbell tumor. Patients usually present with nerve root pain.

Intramedullary tumors are usually astrocytomas and ependymomas. It is important that these intrathecal tumors are differentiated from syringomyelia because both types of tumors present with sensory loss.

DDx

Cervical spondylotic myelopathy, acute cervical disc protrusion, spinal angioma, acute transverse myelitis.

Physical Examination

Patients with tumors of the spine typically present with complaints indicative of progressive spinal cord compression with evidence of a sensory level.

Diagnostic Evaluation

Plain radiographs may demonstrate bony erosion or vertebral body collapse. CT with myelography and MRI are the modalities of choice because they provide detailed anatomic definition. MRI is most helpful in demonstrating intramedullary cord tumors.

Treatment

The goal of spinal tumor treatment is to relieve cord compression and to maintain spinal stability. These are interrelated goals because the removal of a compressing tumor usually requires surgery on the bony spine.

The spine consists of two columns: the anterior column (vertebral bodies, discs and ligaments) and the posterior column (facet joints, neural arch and ligaments). Damage sustained to one of the columns may result in permanent spinal instability.

For anterior tumors that involve the vertebral body, tumor removal via the anterior approach is performed. The vertebral body is resected and the defect repaired with a bone graft, acrylic, or metal hardware.

Posterior tumors can be removed by laminectomy that generally does not cause spinal instability. Laminectomy should not be performed for extradural tumors causing vertebral body collapse because gross spinal instability will result. Metastatic and unresectable disease can be palliated and pain controlled with radiation therapy.

Key Points

Spinal tumors

1. Are either extradural, intradural, or intramedullary;

2. Most extradural tumors are metastatic lesions;

3. Symptoms of progressive spinal cord compression with evidence of a sensory level are typical;

4. Anterior and posterior surgical approaches are utilized.

▶ SPONDYLOSIS AND DISC HERNIATION

Degenerative changes in the spine are responsible for a large proportion of spine disease. Intervertebral discs consist of two parts: the central nucleus pulposus, which acts as a "ball-bearing" between vertebrae, and the surrounding dense anulus fibrosus (Fig. 13-8). At birth, the nucleus contains 80% water, but by age 20, it begins to dehydrate and disc space narrowing occurs. In the cervical and lumbar spines, disc space narrowing causes abnormal vertebral stresses and movement, which in turn causes osteogenesis with the formation of osteophytes and bony spurs. These degenerative bone growths can traumatize nerve roots of the spinal cord itself. This degenerative process secondary to abnormal motion in an aging spine is called spondylosis.

Structural failure of the intervertebral disc occurs when the nucleus pulposus herniates into the spinal canal or neural foramina, through a defect in the circumferential disc anulus. Disc herniation is generally lateral, causing nerve-root compression and radicular symptoms.

These two interrelated degenerative processes are responsible for most spine disease, manifested by nerve root and spinal cord compression. The most mobile segments of the spine (cervical and lumbar) are commonly affected by both processes. Spondylosis is

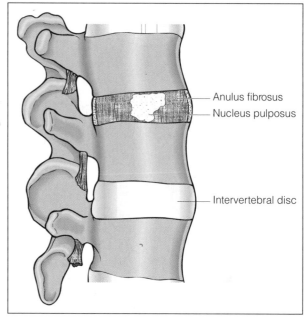

Figure 13-8 Intervertebral disc: anulus fibrosus and centrally located nucleus pulposus.

more common in the cervical region, whereas disc protrusion and prolapse predominates in the lumbar spine (Fig. 13-9).

History

Patients with cervical spondylosis and disc disease are typically older than 50 years and present with complaints of pain, paresthesias, and dysesthesias in cervical dermatomes. In the case of cervical spondylotic myelopathy, secondary to repetitive spinal cord damage by osteophytes, patients experience progressive numbness, weakness, and paresthesias of the hands and forearm in a glove-like distribution. In contradistinction, patients with radiculopathy secondary to disc disease complain of pain radiating down the arm in a nerve-root distribution, worsening on neck extension. Dermatomal weakness, numbness, and tingling often occur in C6 and C7 distributions because these nerve roots pass via the most mobile joints of the spine.

Physical Examination

Limitation of neck motion and straightening of the normal cervical lordosis are common findings. Sensory and motor deficits in a nerve root or glove-like distribution are typical, depending on the focus and mechanism of neuronal injury. Careful testing for signs of diminished bicep and tricep reflexes will afford accurate localization.

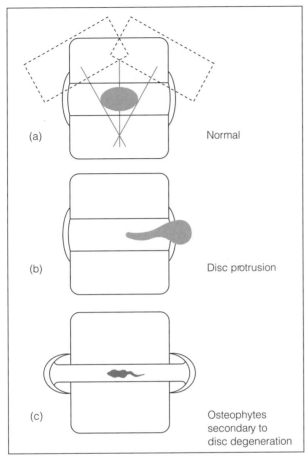

(a) Normal

(b) Disc protrusion

(c) Osteophytes
secondary to
disc degeneration

Figure 13-9 Diagram (a) shows normal disc space with normal rotatory movement of one vertebra upon the adjacent one. Diagram (b) shows a disc protrusion while diagram (c) shows osteophytes developing secondary to disc degeneration (or disc protrusion). Note the different origin of the disc protrusion and osteophytes.

DDx

All causes of cervical spinal cord or cervical nerve root compression must be considered. More common causes of cord compression are rheumatoid arthritis and ankylosing spondylitis. Causes of nerve root compression include cervical rib and scalenus anticus syndromes, carpal tunnel syndrome, ulnar nerve palsy, Pancoast tumor of the pulmonary apex, or a primary CNS tumor of the brachial plexus.

Diagnostic Evaluation

Plain cervical spine films show straightening of the normal cervical lordosis, disc space narrowing, osteophyte formation, and spinal canal narrowing. If the sagittal diameter of the cervical spinal canal is 10 mm or less, clinical manifestations of spinal cord compression are expected.

CT myelography and MRI are used to evaluate the spinal cord and nerve roots and define their relationships to other vertebral structures. Areas of cord and root compression can be identified and intervention planned. MRI is the study of choice for initial evaluation of a herniated cervical disc, whereas CT is preferred when more bony detail is required.

Treatment

All patients should be managed initially with medical therapy except for those with evidence of spinal or foraminal compression. Neck immobilization, cervical traction, analgesics, and muscle relaxants are used. For acute cervical radiculopathy due to cervical disc herniation, over 95% of patients improve without surgery. However, those patients with spondylosis and disc prolapse who fail to improve or exhibit progressive worsening require surgical treatment.

Because the pathogenesis of degenerative osteogenesis is abnormal stress and movement between vertebrae, procedures aimed at stabilizing the spine have shown significant success in obtaining symptomatic relief and promoting osteophyte reabsorption. Anterior cervical fusion produces immobilization by internal fixation and removal of the intervertebral disc with bone graft replacement. Both cervical spondylosis and cervical disc prolapse can be treated with this procedure.

Decompression laminectomy is usually only performed on patients with a diffusely narrow spinal canal who are rapidly worsening due to spondylotic myelopathy. The disadvantage of this approach is that osteophytes continue to progress after posterior decompression.

Lumbar Disc Disease

Lumbar disc prolapse is a common disorder that often presents as pain radiation down the lower extremity to below the knee.

Physical Examination

Symptoms of sciatica are caused by disc herniation lateral to the posterior longitudinal ligament with compression of a nerve root, leading to severe radicular pain. The L4–L5 and L5–S1 discs most commonly prolapse, leading to L5 and S1 nerve-root symptoms. Paresthesia, numbness, and weakness may be present. Straight leg raise testing is positive for pain radiating down the affected extremity with both ipsilateral and contralateral leg raising. Other important signs indicating disc herniation include absence of an ankle reflex, weakness of foot dorsiflexion, and tenderness over the affected spinal disc and nerve root.

Diagnosis

Clinical diagnosis is confirmed by MRI that demonstrates disc protrusion at the suspected level (Fig. 13-10).

Treatment

As most patients improve without surgery, the indication for elective surgery is chronic disabling pain. The standard procedure of choice is open laminectomy and discectomy of the appropriate interspace. Urgent surgery is indicated in patients with progressive neurologic deficits (e.g., foot drop) and in those with acute onset of cauda equina syndrome (CES), which is a neurosurgical emergency and occurs due to a massive midline disc protrusion that compresses the cauda equina. Typical findings of CES include urinary retention, bilateral sciatica, and perineal numbness and tingling. Urgent bilateral laminectomy decompression with disc removal is required.

Key Points

1. Spondylosis and disc herniation present as nerve-root and spinal cord compression.

2. Spondylosis is more common in the cervical region, whereas disc disease predominates in the lumbar spine.

3. Cauda equina syndrome presents as urinary retention, bilateral sciatica, and perineal numbness secondary to massive lumbar disc herniation. Urgent decompressive laminectomy is indicated.

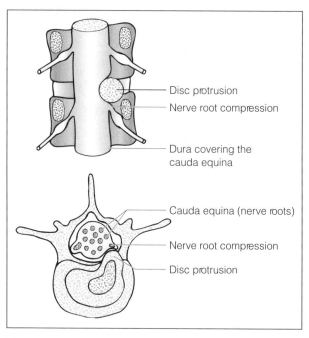

Figure 13-10 Diagram showing the relations of a lumbar disc prolapse. Protruding disk causes nerve root compression.

CHAPTER 14

Organ Transplantation

▸ IMMUNOLOGY

The development of organ transplantation has been a remarkable medical and surgical accomplishment. With advances in immunology and the use of immunosuppressive drugs, the transplantation of the kidney, heart, and liver are now commonplace. With further knowledge and experience, other types of organ transplantation (pancreas, intestine) will be possible.

The key to successful organ transplantation is the ability to control the immunologic reaction when a donor's tissues are rejected by the recipient's body. This host response to the donor's major histocompatibility antigens is the key impediment to organ transplantation.

Major histocompatibility antigens are coded by a single chromosomal complex called the major histocompatibility complex (MHC). In humans, the MHC is named the HLA antigen (human leukocyte antigen) and it is found on the short arm of chromosome 6.

HLA antigens are classified according to their structure and function. Class I antigens are present on virtually all nucleated cells in the human body and act as targets for cytotoxic T cells. Class II antigens are located only on B cells, monocytes, macrophages, and activated T cells and are important in antigen presentation.

The rejection reaction of a transplant recipient directed against mismatched donor HLA antigens is a complex event that involves the actions of cytotoxic T cells, activated T-helper cells, B lymphocytes, activated macrophages, and antibodies. The reaction is primarily cellular in nature and is T-cell dependent. Class I antigens stimulate cytotoxic T cells, which directly causes donor tissue destruction. Class II antigens activate T-helper cells that, along with activated cytotoxic T cells, elaborate interleukin-1 (IL-1) and IL-2 that further activates macrophages and antibody releasing B cells.

Although tissue rejection is primarily a function of cellular immunity, humoral responses are responsible for hyperacute rejection reactions. Donor class I antigens are capable of inciting a hyperacute rejection reaction if cytotoxic antibodies against class I antigens are present in the recipient's serum at the time of transplant. If prior sensitization has occurred through blood transfusions, pregnancy, or earlier transplants, immediate fixation of antibodies to the donor vascular epithelium will result in the formation of platelet and fibrin plugs, with eventual ischemic necrosis of the graft.

Preoperative HLA histocompatibility testing attempts to create a donor-recipient match with the least amount of genetic dissimilarity, thereby reducing the chance of postoperative rejection. When donor and recipient are identical twins (isograft), there is no antigenic difference between individuals. The next closest match is between parents, offspring, and half of siblings, because they all have one identical chromosome. Transplants between nonidentical humans are called allografts. Interspecies transplants are xenografts (Table 14-1).

To avoid hyperacute rejection, cross-matching of the recipient's serum against the donor's lymphocytes is necessary to confirm the presence of pre-existing antibodies against donor tissue antigens. Finally, there must be ABO blood group compatibility between donor and recipient.

▸ IMMUNOSUPPRESSION

Organ transplantation made significant advances in the 1960s with the development of immunosuppressive agents that could control or prevent the rejection reaction. With improved understanding of the immune system, further techniques have been developed to manipulate the rejection process. As the rejection phenomenon varies between different organ transplants, organ-specific immunosuppressive regimens have been developed.

To prevent graft rejection, immunosuppressive agents generally function either to reduce the number of circulating lymphocytes capable of inciting a rejection reaction or to interrupt the antigen-induced lymphocyte response that causes graft rejection.

Agents that induce lymphocyte depletion include antilymphocyte globulin (ALG), monoclonal antibodies (OKT3), radiation, and corticosteroids (prednisone). The destructive capability of ALG appears to be directed mainly against T cells, whereas OKT3 opsonizes

TABLE 14-1

Classification of Graft Types

Graft Type	Relationship of Graft Donor and Recipient
Autograft	Same individual
Isograft	Same species and genetically identical (monozygotic twin)
Allograft	Same species but not genetically identical
Xenograft	Different species

TABLE 14-2

Classification Criteria for Allograft Rejection Responses

Type	Time Course	Target	Response
Hyperacute	Minutes to hours	Vessels	Humoral
Acute	Early after transplant	Parenchyma/vessels	Cellular/humoral
Chronic	Late after transplant	Parenchyma/vessels	Cellular/humoral

T cells that are eventually removed from circulation by reticuloendothelial cells. Prednisone is an inhibitor of both cell-mediated and humoral immunity that decreases the number of circulating lymphocytes by redistributing them to lymphoid tissues and by inhibiting the production of T-cell lymphokines, such as IL-2.

Antiproliferative agents that interrupt the rejection response include azathioprine (Imuran) and cyclosporine (Sandimmune). Azathioprine is a mercaptopurine and antimetabolite that inhibits nucleic acid synthesis, whereas cyclosporine inhibits the production and release of IL-2, a T-cell growth factor, by T-helper cells. Cyclosporine disrupts the development of the cytotoxic T cells responsible for graft rejection.

▶ ALLOGRAFT REJECTION

Despite the use of agents that induce lymphocyte depletion or interrupt the rejection response, graft rejection may occur either acutely or chronically. Table 14-2 describes general criteria used to classify different allograft rejection responses.

Hyperacute rejection is of very rapid onset that occurs soon after the completion of the graft anastomosis. Preformed cytotoxic antibodies against HLA antigens or ABO blood group antigens produce vasculitis, endothelial necrosis, and thrombosis that results in complete graft destruction in only minutes to hours. Because there is no effective treatment of hyperacute rejection, pretransplant cross-match testing is vitally important for graft survival.

Acute rejection may occur during the first few months after transplantation and is mainly due to cellular mechanisms targeting graft parenchyma and vasculature. Interstitial edema, vasculitis, and mixed cell inflammation are seen microscopically. Clinically, patients present with organ failure. Repeated episodes of acute rejection may occur, and treatment is directed toward lymphocyte-depleting agents such as prednisone, ALG, or OKT3.

Chronic rejection is a late occurrence with slow progressive onset, developing months to years after transplantation. Both parenchyma and vessels are targeted by cellular and humoral mechanisms that cause interstitial fibrosis, sclerotic vascular changes, and secondary ischemic injury. Chronic rejection is difficult to treat and graft loss eventually occurs.

▶ KEY POINTS

1. Control of the host response to donor major histocompatibility antigens is the key to organ transplantation.

2. In humans, the major histocompatibility complex is called the HLA antigen.

3. HLA antigens are either class I or class II antigens.

4. Class I antigens are targets for cytotoxic T cells, whereas class II antigens are important in antigen presentation.

5. Tissue rejection is primarily a function of cellular immunity.

6. Hyperacute rejection is a function of humoral responses to HLA or ABO mismatching.

7. Immunosuppressives are used to control or prevent the rejection reaction.

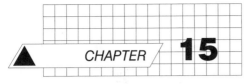

CHAPTER 15

Pancreas

*T*he pancreas is a key regulator of digestion and metabolism through both endocrine and exocrine functions. Intracellular activation of digestive enzymes results in acute and chronic pancreatitis. The most common cause of pancreatitis is alcohol ingestion.

▶ EMBRYOLOGY

Formation of the pancreas begins during the first few weeks of gestation with the development of the ventral and dorsal pancreatic buds. The dorsal bud arises directly from the duodenal endoderm, whereas the ventral bud forms from the endoderm of the hepatic diverticulum and is therefore associated with the developing common bile duct. As development proceeds, the ventral bud migrates dorsally by clockwise rotation and fuses with the larger dorsal bud (Fig. 15-1).

The resulting gland is composed of the uncinate process and inferior pancreatic head, derived from the ventral bud, and the superior head, neck, body and tail, derived from the dorsal bud. The ducts of both buds fuse to create the main pancreatic duct, the duct of Wirsung. Occasionally, the proximal aspect of the dorsal pancreatic duct fails to completely fuse with the ventral duct, resulting in a duct of Santorini, which drains a portion of the exocrine pancreas through a separate minor duodenal papilla (Fig. 15-2).

Important congenital variants of pancreatic development include pancreas divisum, which results in complete failure of dorsal and ventral duct fusion, and annular pancreas, which arises from failure of rotation by the ventral bud resulting in pancreatic tissue completely or partially encircling the second portion of the duodenum. Pancreas divisum has been implicated as a cause of pancreatitis when associated with a relatively stenotic minor duodenal papilla. Annular pancreas has been shown to cause varying degrees of duodenal obstruction, requiring operation in some cases.

▶ ANATOMY AND PHYSIOLOGY

The pancreas is a retroperitoneal structure located posterior to the stomach and anterior to the inferior vena cava and aorta. The yellowish multilobulated gland is divided into four portions: the head, which includes the uncinate process; neck; body; and tail (Fig. 15-3). It lies in a transverse orientation with the pancreatic head in intimate association with the C loop of the duodenum, the body draped over the spine, and the tail nestled in the splenic hilum.

The arterial blood supply to the pancreatic head is derived from parallel anterior and posterior pancreaticoduodenal arteries (Fig. 15-4). These arteries arise from the superior pancreaticoduodenal artery, which is a continuation of the gastroduodenal artery, and from the inferior pancreaticoduodenal artery, which arises from the superior mesenteric artery. The body and tail are supplied from branches of the splenic and left gastroepiploic arteries. Venous drainage follows arterial anatomy and enters the portal circulation.

Both sympathetic and parasympathetic fibers innervate the pancreas. Sympathetic fibers are responsible for transmitting pain of pancreatic origin, whereas efferent postganglionic parasympathetic fibers innervate islet, acini, and ductal systems. In patients with intractable pain from chronic pancreatitis, splanchnicectomy can be performed to interrupt sympathetic pain fibers.

The pancreas is unusual because it is both an endocrine and exocrine organ. In these capacities, it serves many important functions as a principal regulator of nutrient digestion and metabolism.

The functional units of the endocrine pancreas are the islets of Langerhans. The islets are multiple small endocrine glands scattered throughout the pancreas and comprise only 1% to 2% of the total pancreatic cell mass. The bulk of the pancreatic parenchyma is exocrine tissue. Four islet cell types have been identified: A cell (alpha), B cell (beta), D cell (delta), and F cells (PP cell).

The alpha cell produces glucagon, which is secreted in response to stimulation by amino acids, cholecystokinin (CCK), gastrin, catecholamines, and sympathetic and parasympathetic nerves. Its role is to ensure an ample supply of circulating nutritional fuel during periods of fasting. The major site of action is the liver, where it promotes hepatic gluconeogenesis and glycogenolysis, leading to hyperglycemia. Glucagon also inhibits gastrointestinal motility and gastric acid secretion.

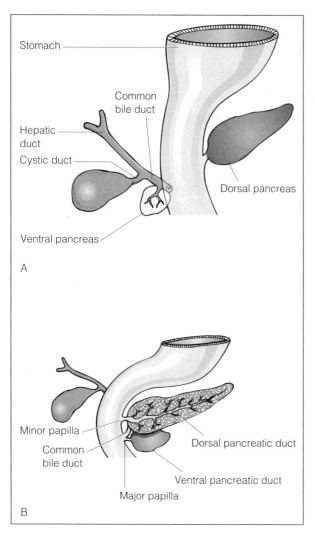

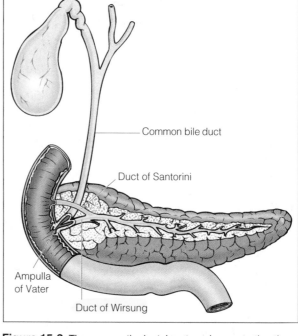

Figure 15-1 After clockwise rotation in a dorsal direction, the ventral pancreas comes to be adjacent to the dorsal pancreas. The dorsal pancreatic duct enters the duodenum at the minor papilla and the ventral pancreatic duct at the major papilla.

Figure 15-2 The pancreatic ductal system demonstrating the ducts of Wirsung (major duct) and Santorini (minor duct).

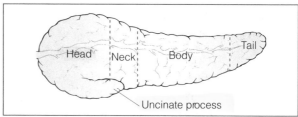

Figure 15-3 Regional anatomy of the pancreas.

The largest percentage of islet volume is occupied by the insulin-producing beta cells. The main function of insulin is to promote the storage of ingested nutrients. Insulin is released into the portal circulation in response to glucose, amino acids, and vagal stimulation. Above all, glucose is the most potent stimulus of insulin release. Insulin has both local and distant anabolic and anticatabolic activity. Local paracrine function is the inhibition of glucagon secretion by alpha cells. In the liver, insulin inhibits gluconeogenesis and promotes the synthesis and storage of glycogen and prevents its breakdown. In adipose tissue, insulin increases glucose uptake by adipocytes, promotes tri-

glyceride storage, and inhibits lipolysis. In muscle, it promotes the synthesis of glycogen and protein.

Somatostatin is secreted by islet delta cells in response to the same stimuli that promote insulin release. Although found in other tissues (brain, intestine), the role of pancreatic somatostatin is to slow the movement of nutrients from the intestine into the circulation. This is achieved by decreasing pancreatic exocrine function, reducing splanchnic blood flow, decreasing gastrin and gastric acid production, and reducing gastric emptying time. Somatostatin also has paracrine inhibitory effects on insulin, glucagon, and pancreatic polypeptide (PP) secretion.

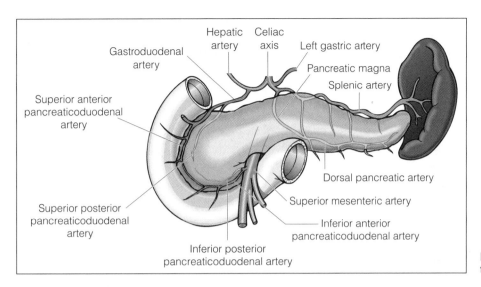

Figure 15-4 Blood supply of the pancreas.

F cells secrete PP after ingestion of a mixed meal. The function of PP is unknown; however, it may be important in "priming" hepatocytes for gluconeogenesis. Patients with pancreatic endocrine tumors have been noted to have elevated levels of circulating PP.

The basic functional unit of the exocrine pancreas is the acinus. Each acinus is comprised of a single layer of acinar cells arranged in circular formation. Acinar cells contain zymogen granules in the apical region of the cytoplasm. Acini are drained by a converging ductal system that terminates in the main pancreatic ex-

cretory duct. The centroacinar cells of individual acini form the origins of the ducts, with intercalated duct cells lining the remainder (Fig. 15-5).

Exocrine pancreatic secretions are products of both ductal and acinar cells. Ductal cells contribute a clear, basic pH, isotonic solution of water and electrolytes, rich in bicarbonate ions. Secretion of pancreatic fluid is principally controlled by secretin, a hormone produced in the mucosal S cells of the crypts of Lieberkuhn in the proximal small bowel. The presence of intraluminal acid and bile stimulates secretin release, which binds pancreatic ductal cell receptors causing fluid secretion.

Pancreatic digestive enzymes are synthesized by and excreted from acinar cells. Proenzymes are packaged into zymogen granules that are stored in the apical portion of the acinar cell. After acinar cell stimulation by secretagogues (CCK, acetylcholine), the zymogen granules fuse with the apical cell membrane and are extruded into the centroacinar luminal space via exocytosis. Enzymes that are excreted include the endopeptidases (trypsinogen, chymotrypsinogen, and proelastase) and the exopeptidases (procarboxypeptidase A and B). Other enzymes produced are amylase, lipase, and colipase. All peptidases are excreted into the ductal system as inactive precursors. Once in the duodenum, trypsinogen is converted to the active form, trypsin, by interaction with duodenal mucosal enterokinase. Trypsin, in turn, serves to then activate the other excreted peptidases. In contrast to the peptidases, the enzymes amylase and lipase are excreted into the ductal system in their active forms (Fig. 15-6).

Figure 15-5 Cellular structure of a pancreatic acinus.

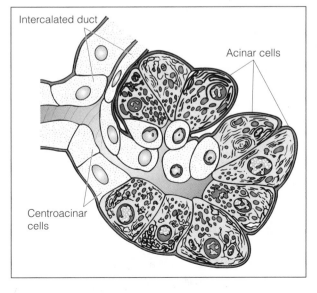

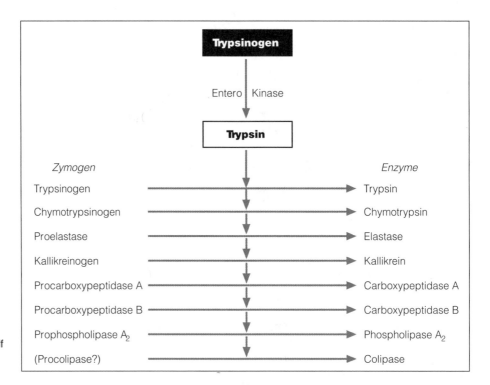

Figure 15-6 Activation of pancreatic enzymes from the action of trypsin, which is itself activated by the action of enterokinase.

▶ KEY POINTS

1. The pancreas is a retroperitoneal structure consisting of a head, neck, body, and tail.

2. The duct of Wirsung drains the mature pancreas. Occasionally, a duct of Santorini drains through a separate minor papilla.

3. Congenital variants arise from aberrant pancreatic bud migration.

4. The islets of Langerhans of the endocrine pancreas include alpha cells (glucagon), beta cells (insulin), delta cells (somatostatin), and PP cells (pancreatic polypeptide).

5. Trypsinogen is converted to trypsin by duodenal mucosal enterokinase.

6. Trypsin then activates the other excreted peptidases.

▶ ACUTE PANCREATITIS
Pathogenesis

Acute pancreatitis is a disease of glandular enzymatic autodigestion with varying presentations ranging from mild parenchymal edema to life-threatening hemorrhagic pancreatitis. Multiple etiologies have been identified, with alcoholism and biliary tract disease accounting for 80% to 90% of cases. The remainder of cases are attributed to hypertriglyceridemia, hy-

TABLE 15-1
Causes of Acute Pancreatitis
Alcohol
Biliary tract disease
Hyperlipidemia
Hypercalcemia
Familial
Trauma—external, operative, ERCP
Ischemic—hypotension, cardiopulmonary bypass
Pancreatic duct obstruction—tumor, pancreas divisum, ampullary stenosis, ascaris infestation
Duodenal obstruction
Infection—mycoplasma, mumps, Coxsackie

percalcemia, trauma, infection, ischemia, endoscopic retrograde cholangiopancreatography (ERCP), and cardiopulmonary bypass (Table 15-1). The exact pathogenesis of acute pancreatitis remains unclear; however, obstruction of the ampulla of Vater by gallstones, spasm, or edema is thought to cause elevated intraductal pressure and bile reflux into the pancreatic duct. The final common pathway is the activation and extravasation of intraparenchymal enzymes, resulting in tissue destruction and ischemic necrosis of the pancreas and retroperitoneal tissues.

History

Because of the different degrees of pancreatic tissue destruction seen in cases of pancreatitis, the presentation of acute disease is varied and diagnosis may be difficult. Important past medical history includes information regarding prior episodes of pancreatitis, alcoholism, and biliary colic. Patients usually present with complaints of upper abdominal pain, often radiating to the back, nausea, vomiting, and a low-grade fever. A severe attack of pancreatitis is manifest by hypotension, sepsis, and multiorgan failure. Patients with an alcoholic etiology usually experience pain 12 to 48 hours after alcohol ingestion. Gallstone pancreatitis presents with a more acute onset, often after a large meal.

Patients have upper abdominal tenderness, usually without peritoneal signs. The abdomen may be slightly distended secondary to a paralytic ileus. Fever and tachycardia are common.

DDx

Acute pancreatitis is often difficult to differentiate from other causes of upper abdominal pain. The clinical presentation may mimic that of a perforated peptic ulcer or acute biliary tract disease. Other conditions that may have similar presentations are acute intestinal obstruction, acute mesenteric thrombosis, and a leaking abdominal aortic aneurysm.

Diagnostic Evaluation

Over 90% of patients presenting with acute pancreatitis have an elevated serum amylase. However, amylase levels are relatively nonspecific because many other intra-abdominal conditions cause amylase elevation. Such conditions include intestinal obstruction, perforated peptic ulcer, and biliary tract disease. If the diagnosis is unclear, a lipase level should also be measured because it is solely of pancreatic origin.

Leukocytosis greater than 10,000 is common, and hemoconcentration with azotemia may also be present because of significant third-space fluid sequestration. Hyperglycemia frequently occurs due to hypoinsulinemia, and hypocalcemia occurs from calcium deposition in areas of fat necrosis.

Routine chest x-ray may reveal a left pleural effusion, known as a "sympathetic effusion," secondary to peripancreatic inflammation. Air under the diaphragm indicates perforation of a hollow viscus, such as a perforated peptic ulcer.

The classic radiographic finding on abdominal plain films is a "sentinel loop" of dilated mid- to distal duodenum or proximal jejunum located in the left upper quadrant, adjacent to the inflamed pancreas. Similarly, the "colon cutoff sign" is a distended transverse colon with an airless distal colon beyond the splenic flexure. In cases of gallstone pancreatitis, radiopaque densities are usually seen in the right upper quadrant.

CT is the most sensitive radiologic study for confirming the diagnosis of acute pancreatitis. Virtually all patients show evidence of either parenchymal or peripancreatic changes. CT is also of great use in defining the subsequent complications of pancreatitis, such as phlegmon or pseudocyst formation. CT-guided interventional techniques may also be performed to drain peripancreatic fluid collections to rule out infection or for treatment.

Because the clinical course of pancreatitis can vary from mild inflammation to fatal hemorrhagic disease, prompt identification of patients at risk for developing complications may improve final outcomes. Ranson's criteria are well-known prognostic signs used for predicting the severity of disease (Table 15-2). The ability to predict a patient's course at the time of admission and over the initial 48 hours allows appropriate therapy to be instituted early in the hospitalization. Mortality rates correlate with the number of criteria present at admission and during the initial 48 hours after admission: 0 to 2 criteria, 1% mortality; 3 to 4, 16%; 5 to 6, 40%; and 7 to 8, 100%.

Treatment

Medical treatment of pancreatitis involves supportive care of the patient and treatment of complications as they arise. No effective agent exists to reverse the inflammatory response initiated by the activated zymogens. However, with adequate care, most cases are self-limited and resolve spontaneously.

Hydration is the most important early intervention in treating acute pancreatitis because significant third-spacing occurs secondary to parenchymal and retroperitoneal inflammation. Hypovolemia must be

TABLE 15-2

Ranson's Criteria for Acute Pancreatitis

At Admission	During Initial 48 Hours
Age > 55	Hematocrit fall > 10 percent
White blood cell count > 16,000	Blood urea nitrogen rise > 5
Serum glucose > 200	Calcium fall to < 8
Serum LDH > 350	Arterial PO_2 < 60
SGOT > 250	Base deficit > 4
	Fluid sequestration > 6 liters

avoided because pancreatic ischemia may quickly develop secondary to inadequate splanchnic blood flow.

Traditional treatment calls for putting the pancreas "to rest" by not feeding the patient. The goal is to decrease pancreatic stimulation, thereby suppressing pancreatic exocrine function. Nasogastric suction may be instituted to treat symptoms of nausea and vomiting.

If the severity of disease necessitates the patient to stop oral intake for a prolonged period, then an alternative method of administering nutrition must be instituted. Intravenous nutrition (total parenteral nutrition/hyperalimentation) is commonly given. Once an attack resolves, gradual advancement of oral intake proceeds, beginning with low fat liquids high in carbohydrates to avoid pancreatic stimulation.

Oxygen therapy may be necessary for treatment of hypoxia, which often occurs secondary to pulmonary changes thought to be due to circulating mediators. The degree of hypoxia is directly related to the severity of pancreatic inflammation. Evidence of atelectasis, pleural effusion, pulmonary edema, and adult respiratory distress syndrome may be seen on chest radiograph.

Surgical treatment of acute pancreatitis is directed at complications that develop secondary to the underlying disease process. During the early phase of pancreatitis, a phlegmon with areas of necrosis may form because of inflammation and edema caused by tissue ischemia and enzyme activation. Necrotic areas will eventually liquefy and are at risk for infection if they are unable to reabsorb and heal. Large collections, not resolving as demonstrated by serial CTs, require surgical debridement and drainage to avoid fatal septic complications.

Peripancreatic collections that persist after the inflammatory phase has subsided may develop a thickened wall or "rind." Such collections are called pancreatic pseudocysts. Drainage is usually required for cysts greater than 6 cm in diameter that have persisted for more than 6 weeks to alleviate symptoms or prevent major complications. Standard therapy is internal drainage into the stomach, duodenum, or small intestine. The most easy and effective procedure is cyst gastrostomy, where the mature cyst is drained through the adherent posterior stomach wall.

During the later stage of disease, abscess formation may occur. The pathogenesis is a progression: an ischemic parenchyma becomes necrotic and liquefies, forming a fluid collection seeded by bacteria that eventually progresses to abscess formation. Most bacteria are of enteric origin, and standard antibiotic therapy is insufficient treatment. Proper treatment requires adherence to the surgical adage: "all pus must be drained for healing to occur." If surgical drainage and debridement is not performed, the mortality rate is 100%. Percutaneous drainage is usually not adequate because only the fluid component is removed and the necrotic tissue remains.

Hemorrhage secondary to erosion of blood vessels by activated proteases can be a life-threatening complication. Often it is the main hepatic or splenic artery that bleeds. If control is not achieved angiographically, then surgical exploration is required.

Key Points

Acute pancreatitis

1. Is mostly caused by alcohol and biliary tract disease in Western populations;

2. Results from glandular autodigestion caused by intraparenchymal enzyme activation;

3. Uses Ranson's criteria to predict the severity of disease and estimate mortality;

4. Is usually self-limiting and resolves spontaneously with supportive care;

5. Is treated surgically for such complications as phlegmon, pseudocyst, abscess, or hemorrhage.

▶ CHRONIC PANCREATITIS

Of patients with acute pancreatitis, a very small number will progress to develop chronic pancreatitis. The chronic form of disease is characterized by persistent inflammation that causes destructive fibrosis of the gland. The clinical picture is of recurring or persistent upper abdominal pain with evidence of malabsorption, steatorrhea, and diabetes.

Pathogenesis

Chronic pancreatitis can be divided into two forms: calcific pancreatitis, usually associated with persistent alcohol abuse, and obstructive pancreatitis, secondary to pancreatic duct obstruction before the onset of disease.

Alcohol-induced calcific pancreatitis is the most common form of disease in Western populations. Proposed mechanisms of disease include ductal plugging and occlusion by protein and mineral precipitates. The resulting inflammation and patchy fibrosis subsequently leads to parenchymal destruction and eventual atrophy of the gland.

Obstructive chronic pancreatitis is due to ductal blockage secondary to scarring from acute pancreatitis or trauma, papillary stenosis, pseudocyst, or tumor, which results in upstream duct dilatation and inflammation.

History

Abdominal pain is the principal presenting complaint and the most frequent indication for surgery. The pain is upper abdominal, either intermittent or persistent, and frequently radiates to the back. Patients are often addicted to narcotic pain relievers. Other symptoms result from exocrine insufficiency (malabsorption) and endocrine insufficiency (diabetes mellitus).

Diagnostic Evaluation

The diagnosis of chronic pancreatitis is best made using imaging techniques that detect pancreatic morphologic changes rather than tests of glandular function, given the functional reserve of the pancreas. The best test of exocrine function is the secretin-cholecystokinin test which is now rarely used.

The radiologic signs of chronic pancreatitis include a heterogeneously inflamed or atrophied gland, a dilated and strictured pancreatic duct, and the presence of calculi. Ultrasonography and CT are useful initial imaging procedures; however, ERCP is the most accurate means of diagnosing chronic pancreatitis, because it clearly defines the pancreatic ductal system and the biliary tree.

Treatment

The effective treatment of chronic abdominal pain is often the focus of care for patients with chronic pancreatitis. Opiates are very useful for controlling visceral pain; however, many patients become opiate-dependent over the long term. Alcohol nerve blocks of the celiac plexus have only moderate success.

Pancreatic exocrine insufficiency is treated with oral pancreatic enzymes and insulin is used to treat diabetes mellitus, if present. Ethanol intake by the patient must cease.

Surgical intervention is undertaken only if medical therapy has proven unsuccessful in relieving chronic intractable pain. Functional drainage of the pancreatic duct and the resection of diseased tissue are the goals of any procedure. Based on ERCP and CT findings, the correct operation can be planned.

For patients with a "chain of lakes" appearing pancreatic duct caused by sequential ductal scarring and dilatation, a longitudinal pancreaticojejunostomy (Puestow procedure) is indicated to achieve adequate drainage. A Roux-en-Y segment of proximal jejunum is anastomosed side-to-side with the opened pancreatic duct facilitating drainage (Fig. 15-7).

Distal pancreatic duct obstruction with associated parenchymal disease is best treated by performing a distal pancreatectomy (Du Vale procedure).

Key Points

In chronic pancreatitis,

1. Alcohol use is the most common cause;
2. Exocrine insufficiency (malabsorption) and endocrine insufficiency (diabetes mellitus) may occur;
3. Surgical treatment includes longitudinal pancreaticojejunostomy (Puestow procedure) or distal pancreatectomy (Du Vale procedure).

▶ PANCREATIC CANCER

Epidemiology

Pancreatic adenocarcinoma is a leading cause of cancer death, trailing other cancers such as lung and colon. Men are affected more than women by a 2:1 ratio. Risk factors for developing pancreatic cancer are increasing age and cigarette smoking. The peak incidence is in the fifth and sixth decades. Ductal adenocarcinoma accounts for 80% of the cancer types and is usually found in the head of the gland. Local spread to contiguous structures occurs early and metastases to regional lymph nodes and liver follow.

History

The signs and symptoms of carcinoma of the head of the pancreas are intrinsically related to the regional anatomy of the gland. Patients classically present complaining of obstructive jaundice, weight loss, and constant deep abdominal pain due to peripancreatic tumor infiltration. About half of patients present with jaundice and a palpable nontender gallbladder indicating tumor obstruction of the common bile duct (Courvoiser's Law). Pruritus often accompanies the development of jaundice.

DDx

Carcinoma of the ampulla of Vater, distal common bile duct, or duodenum.

Diagnostic Evaluation

The most common laboratory abnormalities are elevated alkaline phosphatase and direct bilirubin levels, indicating obstructive jaundice. The average bilirubin level in neoplastic obstruction is 18 mg/mL, which is much higher than that seen in gallstone disease. Stool specimens are positive for occult blood in about half of cases.

CT and ERCP are the modalities of choice for the workup of pancreatic cancer. CT reveals the location of the mass, evidence of tumor invasion, and the degree of ductal dilatation. ERCP defines the ductal anatomy and assesses the extent of ductal obstruction. Biopsy

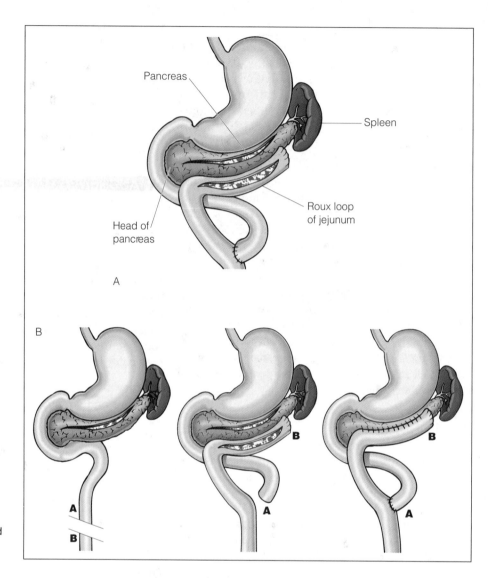

Figure 15-7 Longitudinal pancreaticojejunostomy used in the treatment of chronic pancreatitis.

specimens can be obtained at endoscopy for confirmatory tissue diagnosis.

Imaging information suggesting unresectability includes local tumor extension, contiguous organ invasion, superior mesenteric artery (SMA) or portal vessel invasion, ascites, and distant metastases.

Treatment

The operation for resectable tumors in the head of the pancreas is pancreaticoduodenectomy (Whipple procedure) (Fig. 15-8). This major operation entails the en bloc resection of the antrum, duodenum, proximal jejunum, head of pancreas, gallbladder, and distal common bile duct. A vagotomy is also performed; however, a modified "pylorus sparing" procedure pre-serves the antrum and pylorus, thus obviating the need for vagotomy.

Prognosis

Very few patients are completely cured of their disease, and most die within a year from the time of diagnosis. Among all groups of patients, the 5-year survival for tumors of the head of the pancreas is about 3%. For patients with tumors amenable to Whipple resection, the 5-year survival is 10% to 15%, depending on the node status. Tumors of the body and tail are invariably fatal because diagnosis is made much later due to the lack of obstructive findings.

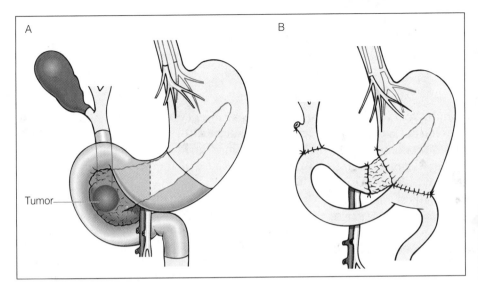

Figure 15-8 Pancreaticoduodenectomy (Whipple procedure). Preoperative anatomic relationships (A) and postoperative reconstruction (B).

Key Points

In pancreatic cancer,

1. Obstructive jaundice, weight loss, and abdominal pain are common findings;

2. Courvoiser's law is jaundice and a nontender palpable gallbladder, indicating tumor obstruction of the common bile duct;

3. Bilirubin levels are typically much higher than in gallstone disease;

4. CT and ERCP are used to determine tumor resectability;

5. Resectable tumors of the head of the pancreas are removed by pancreaticoduodenectomy (Whipple procedure). Prognosis is poor.

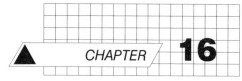

CHAPTER 16

Parathyroid Gland

*7*he surgical treatment of parathyroid disease relates mainly to hyperparathyroidism. Primary hyperparathyroidism results from autonomous parathyroid hormone (PTH) secretion secondary to glandular hyperplasia, parathyroid adenomas, or, rarely, parathyroid carcinoma. Clinical manifestations of disease are caused by persistent hypercalcemia. Fortunately, the surgical removal of hyperfunctioning glands affords a greater than 90% cure rate.

▶ ANATOMY

Parathyroid glands are small yellowish-brown ovals, measuring about 2 × 3 × 5 mm. Normal individuals possess four parathyroid glands; however, five, six, or seven glands are possible. Embryonically, the upper paired glands arise from the fourth branchial pouch and are located behind the thyroid gland, in close association with the inferior thyroid artery (Figs. 16-1 and 16-2). The lower two glands, as well as the thymus, arise from the third branchial pouch and are usually located within 2 cm of the lower thyroid pole (Fig. 16-3). The arterial supply to all four glands is from the inferior thyroid artery.

Aberrant migration may produce ectopic parathyroid glands. Based on their embryologic development, aberrant upper glands are usually intrathyroid or posterior mediastinal, whereas aberrant lower glands are usually intrathymic or anterior mediastinal (Fig. 16-4).

▶ PATHOGENESIS

Several different forms of hyperparathyroidism exist. Primary hyperparathyroidism results from excess PTH, which causes mobilization of calcium deposits from bone, inhibition of renal phosphate reabsorption, and stimulation of renal tubular absorption of calcium. The result is hypercalcemia and hypophosphatemia. Overall, however, both total body calcium and phosphate wasting occur, leading to osteoporosis and bony mineral loss. Such metabolic imbalance leads to the development of associated conditions such as pancreatitis, nephrolithiasis, nephrocalcinosis, gout, pseudogout, hypertension, and peptic ulcer disease.

Secondary hyperparathyroidism is usually seen in patients with renal disease. In renal disease, hyper-

phosphatemia causes depression of serum ionized Ca levels. Hypocalcemia then serves to stimulate excess PTH production by glands that typically have become hyperplastic because of the persistent hypocalcemic stimulus.

Tertiary hyperparathyroidism results from longstanding secondary hyperparathyroidism as persistent hypocalcemia causes the development of autonomous hyperplastic gland function. As in secondary hyperparathyroidism, tertiary disease is seen in dialysis-dependent patients with end-stage renal disease.

Pseudohyperparathyroidism results in a similar biochemical derangement as seen in primary hyperparathyroidism. Oat cell and squamous cell cancers of the lung, head and neck, kidney, and ovary produce

Figure 16-1 Diagram of the pharyngeal pouches. The inferior parathyroid arises from the third pouch and the superior arises from the fourth.

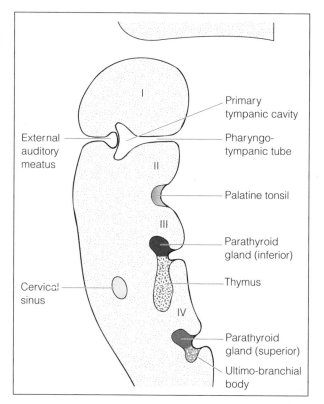

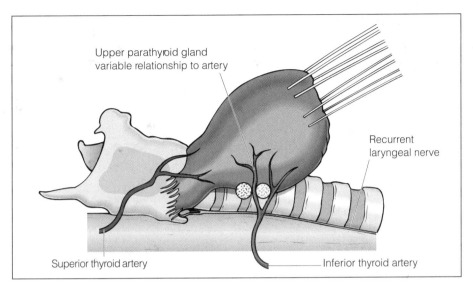

Upper parathyroid gland
variable relationship to artery

Recurrent
laryngeal nerve

Superior thyroid artery

Inferior thyroid artery

Figure 16-2 Normal siting of the upper parathyroid glands.

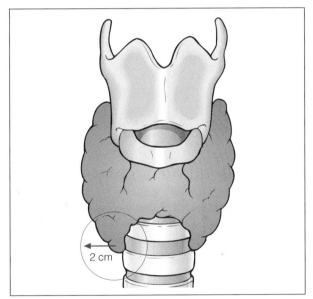

2 cm

Figure 16-3 Normal siting of the lower parathyroid glands.

PTH-like proteins that produce a similar picture of hypercalcemia.

▶ EPIDEMIOLOGY

Hyperparathyroidism is the most common cause of hypercalcemia and has an incidence of 0.1% to 0.3% of the population (Table 16-1). The incidence of disease increases with age, and presentations before puberty are uncommon. Women are affected twice as often as men. Approximately 90% of cases are sporadic and are due to a single hyperfunctioning adenoma. The remainder are of genetic origin as hyperparathyroid-

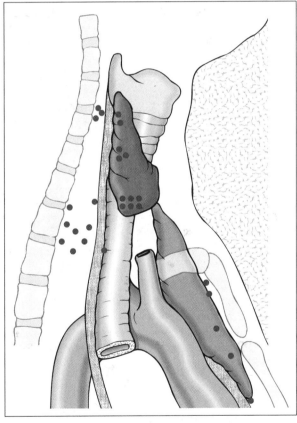

Figure 16-4 Parathyroid gland location after reoperation for persistent hyperparathyroidism.

ism is a component of multiple endocrine neoplastic (MEN) disease. Patients with MEN type I (Wermer's syndrome) have involvement of the three Ps: parathyroid, pituitary, and pancreas. MEN type IIa (Sipple's

TABLE 16-1

Diseases and Factors Causing Hypercalcemia

Hyperparathyroidism
Malignancy
Hyperthyroidism
Multiple myeloma
Sarcoid and other granulomatous diseases
Milk-alkali syndrome
Vitamin D intoxication
Vitamin A intoxication
Paget's disease
Immobilization
Thiazide diuretics
Addisonian crisis
Familial hypocalciuric hypercalcemia

disease) includes hyperparathyroidism, pheochromo-cytoma, and medullary cancer of the thyroid. Patients with MEN I or II have diffuse four gland hyperplasia and require bilateral neck exploration for removal of all affected glands.

▶ RISK FACTORS

Childhood radiation therapy to the head and neck has been proposed as a risk factor for the development of hyperparathyroidism. A family history of MEN is also important.

▶ HISTORY

Historically, patients with primary hyperparathyroidism presented with advanced end-stage renal disease due to staghorn calculi and obstructive uropathy. Pathologic fractures due to bone reabsorption were typical. These days, patients are generally asymptomatic on presentation because diagnosis is usually now made after hypercalcemia is discovered on routine screening. Despite earlier diagnosis, the symptoms of hyperparathyroidism are easily remembered by the time-honored rhyme, "Bones, stones, abdominal groans, psychic moans, and fatigue overtones":

▲ Bones—Aches and arthralgias result from fractures and structural changes in bony architecture. Pseudogout (chondrocalcinosis) causes severe joint pain when articular cartilage becomes calcified.

▲ Stones—Renal calculi from hypercalcemia can produce symptoms of renal colic. Calculi can also cause obstructive uropathy with resulting urinary tract infections and renal failure. Less common is the calcification of the renal parenchyma itself (nephrocalcinosis).

▲ Abdominal groans—Several abdominal conditions can arise from hypercalcemia. The filtration of high serum calcium loads can cause dehydration and subsequent constipation. Pancreatitis can develop secondary to hypercalcemia. Hypercalcemia is also thought to stimulate gastrin production, which leads to elevated gastric acid secretion. Peptic ulcer disease may also be exacerbated.

▲ Psychic moans—Hypercalcemia causes anorexia and associated nausea and vomiting. As with constipation, high mineral levels in the kidney cause polyuria, which leads to thirst and polydipsia. Behavioral changes such as mood swings, organic psychosis, and dementia can be seen.

▲ Fatigue—Hypercalcemia can produce a sense of lassitude and muscular fatigability.

▶ PHYSICAL EXAMINATION

Physical examination is generally unremarkable. Occasionally, a neck mass may be palpable. Rarely, localized aggregates of osteoclasts (osteoclastomas or "brown tumors") can cause focal bone swelling.

▶ DDx

Ectopic tumors, milk alkali syndrome, hyperthyroidism, thiazide diuretics.

▶ DIAGNOSTIC EVALUATION

The most important finding is persistent hypercalcemia, followed by elevated serum PTH levels. Elevated alkaline phosphatase levels indicate bony disease. Renal function is assessed by creatinine measurement.

Bone films may show evidence of subperiosteal reabsorption of the phalanges, osteopenia, osteoclastomas, and metastatic calcifications. Bone densitometry quantifies osteopenia. Abdominal films may reveal renal calculi or nephrocalcinosis.

▶ TREATMENT

Primary hyperparathyroidism is a surgical disease, and operation is required for removal of hyperfunctioning glands. Patients may present in hypercalcemic crisis (coma, delirium, anorexia, vomiting, and abdominal pain) for which vigorous intravenous hydration and forced caluresis with furosemide is the initial therapy. Once the patient is stabilized and the diagnosis of hyperparathyroidism is confirmed, a surgeon may elect to perform preoperative localization of the parathyroid tumor. This can be achieved with ultrasonography, CT, or thallium-technetium scan. For patients undergoing reoperation, selective venous sampling with PTH immunoassay is recommended.

The surgical approach for parathyroid procedures is identical to that used for thyroid disease. Through a curvilinear necklace incision, most tumors are usually found attached to the posterior capsule of the thyroid, overlying the recurrent laryngeal nerve and in close proximity to the inferior thyroid artery. All four glands should be identified because multiple adenomas do occur. In parathyroid hyperplasia, all glands are diseased, which necessitates their surgical removal, except for a single gland, which is subtotally excised. The remaining focus of hyperplastic cells functions to prevent permanent hypocalcemia.

Secondary hyperparathyroidism of renal disease, resulting from low levels of ionized calcium, is treated medically, whereas tertiary hyperparathyroidism, due to autonomous parathyroid hyperplasia, occasionally requires surgical intervention.

After surgery, hypocalcemia occurs secondary to reduced PTH levels and osseous remineralization known as the "hungry bones" phenomenon. Symptoms of hypocalcemia include perioral numbness, paresthesias, carpopedal spasm, and seizures. Chvostek's sign may be elicited by gently tapping the facial nerve causing facial muscle spasm. For mild symptoms of hypocalcemia, treatment consists of oral calcium supplementation and a high-calcium diet. Spasm and seizure activity require immediate treatment with intravenous calcium gluconate or calcium chloride. Recurrent hyperparathyroidism after the removal of a single adenoma occurs in 5% of cases. Attempts at localization should be made with venous sampling and mediastinal imaging. Cervical re-exploration is indicated and sternal split may be necessary.

▶ **KEY POINTS**

1. Hyperparathyroidism is the most common cause of hypercalcemia.

2. Primary hyperparathyroidism results from autonomous PTH secretion by adenomas, hyperplasia, or carcinoma. A single hyperfunctioning adenoma accounts for about 90% of cases.

3. The paired upper glands arise from the fourth branchial pouch and the lower glands and thymus arise from the third branchial pouch. Aberrant migration produces ectopic parathyroid glands.

4. Excess PTH causes bony calcium mobilization, stimulation of renal calcium reabsorption, and inhibition of renal phosphate absorption. Hypercalcemia and hypophosphatemia occur.

5. Primary hyperparathyroidism is associated with pancreatitis, nephrolithiasis, nephrocalcinosis, gout, pseudogout, hypertension, and peptic ulcer disease.

6. Secondary and tertiary hyperparathyroidism occur in patients with renal disease.

7. Pseudohyperparathyroidism occurs in oat cell and squamous carcinomas that produce PTH-like proteins.

8. Hyperparathyroidism occurs in MEN I and MEN IIa.

9. Symptoms of hyperparathyroidism can be remembered by the rhyme "bones, stones, abdominal groans, psychic moans, and fatigue overtones."

10. Postoperative hypocalcemia ("hungry bones" phenomenon) is manifested by periorbital numbness, paresthesias, carpopedal spasm, seizures, and a positive Chvostek's sign.

CHAPTER 17

Skin Cancer

▶ BASAL CELL CARCINOMA

Basal cell carcinoma (BCC) is the most common form of skin cancer in the white population. BCC is rare in Asians and exceedingly rare in blacks. The predominant etiology is excess exposure to ultraviolet B radiation (UVB). Accordingly, BCC is a disease of adults, and tumors arise from sun-exposed skin, namely the head and neck. The cellular origin of BCC has traditionally been thought to be the basal cell of the epidermis. More recently, an alternative theory posits that the originating cell type is a pluripotential epithelial cell. BBC is divided into three types: noduloulcerative, superficial, and sclerosing.

Noduloulcerative BCC

Lesions have a pearly dome-shaped nodular appearance with associated telangiectasia and an ulcerated center. Telangiectasia is secondary to tumor-induced angiogenesis, and ulceration results from outgrowth of the local blood supply. Noduloulcerative lesions are the most common type of basal cell cancer.

Tumors less than 1 cm in diameter are rarely invasive and can be treated with cautery and curettage or cryosurgery. Tumors greater than 1 cm are treated with surgical excision. "High-risk" sites of tumor growth are areas with underlying bone and cartilage (i.e., nose, ear), because the growing tumor tends to track along these structures. Such tumors have a high recurrence rate. Therefore, high-risk tumors and recurrent tumors should be treated with Moh's micrographic surgery to ensure complete excision (Fig. 17-1).

Superficial BCC

The second most common basal cell cancer is the superficial type. Lesions usually appear on the trunk and proximal extremities and clinically resemble thin, scaly, pink plaques with irregular margins (Fig. 17-2). These horizontally expanding tumors often are dismissed as dermatitis, and subsequently, tumors reach diameters of several centimeters by the time of diagnosis. By this late stage, there is ulceration and deep dermal invasion. Standard treatment has been wide-margin excision, with skin grafting if necessary. However, this approach may be unacceptably morbid, leaving a large skin defect. Recently, topical chemotherapy

with 5-FU, cryosurgery, and cautery/curettage have shown cure rates similar to traditional wide excision.

Sclerosing BCC

This is the least common type of basal cell cancer. The anatomic distribution is similar to the noduloulcerative type, but histologically the lesions appear as narrow cords of tumor cells encased in a proliferation of connective tissue. Macroscopically, lesions are smooth, atrophic and indurated, and easily mimic scar tissue. This deceptive appearance is unfortunate because sclerosing tumors are more aggressive than other basal cell tumor types. The growth pattern follows tissue planes and neurovascular bundles, resulting in deep soft tissue invasion. Moh's micrographic surgery is the preferred management technique.

Key Points

Basal cell carcinoma

1. Is the most common form of skin cancer;
2. Is predominantly caused by excess UVB radiation from sunlight;
3. Appears mostly on sun-exposed areas (head and neck);
4. Consists of three types: noduloulcerative, superficial, and sclerosing;
5. Is treated by surgical excision.

▶ MELANOMA

Melanoma is a potentially lethal skin cancer resulting from malignant transformation of the normal melanocyte, usually located in the basal layer of the epidermis.

Pathogenesis

Ultraviolet light is suspected to play a role in the development of all types of skin cancer, including melanoma. Although the precise etiologic role of UV light in the malignant transformation of skin cells remains unresolved, both UVA and UVB are thought to have carcinogenic potential. UVA penetrates deep into the dermis, damaging connective tissue and intrinsic skin elasticity. This aging effect of UVA is balanced by the tanning effect of UVB, because UVB stimulates melanocytes to produce melanin. Excessive UVB exposure results in sunburn.

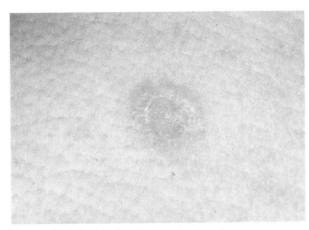

Figure 17-1 Noduloulcerative basal cell carcinoma.

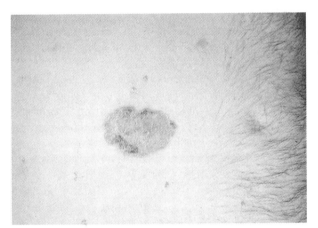

Figure 17-2 Superficial basal cell carcinoma.

Epidemiology

Melanoma accounts for 5% of all skin malignancies and 3% of all cancers. The diagnosis of melanoma carries a 50% mortality in the United States, and the incidence has dramatically increased over the last 10 to 15 years. Most lesions arise from pre-existing moles. A mole showing rapid growth and heterogenous pigmentation should be evaluated and possibly biopsied to rule out melanoma. Fair-skinned individuals have a higher incidence of melanoma than the general population.

Risk Factors

These include a mole showing persistent changes in shape, size, or color; persons having greater than 50 nevi at least 2 mm in diameter; a family history of melanoma; excess sun exposure; immunocompromised status (e.g., immunosuppression, AIDS); and dysplastic nevi in individuals who have two family members with melanoma.

Melanoma Types

Superficial spreading melanoma can occur anywhere, on both sun-exposed and nonexposed areas. The average age of diagnosis is 40 to 50 years. Lesions are commonly on the upper back and on the lower legs. Lesions show heterogeneous pigmentation with irregular margins. The growth phase is radial with horizontal spread (Fig. 17-3).

Lentigo maligna melanoma is usually seen in older individuals; the average age of diagnosis is 70 years. Lesions appear on sun-exposed surfaces, particularly the malar region of the cheek and temple. Lesions exhibit horizontal spread (Fig. 17-4).

Acral lentiginous melanoma has an unusual distribution in that lesions appear on palms, soles, nail beds, or mucous membranes. The most common mucous membrane site is the vulva. Other sites include the anus, nasopharynx, sinuses, and oral cavity. The average age of diagnosis is 60 years. Spread is in a horizontal pattern.

Figure 17-3 Superficial spreading melanoma.

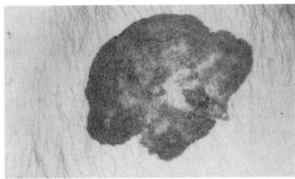

Figure 17-4 Lentigo maligna melanoma.

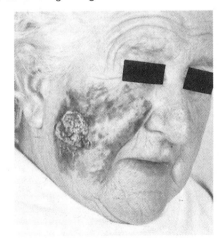

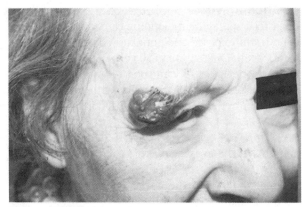

Figure 17-5 Nodular melanoma.

Nodular melanoma can occur at any site and has a very early malignant potential secondary to a predominantly vertical growth phase. In contradistinction, the three other melanoma types exhibit radial growth phases with horizontal spread. Nodular lesions have well-circumscribed borders and uniform black or brown coloring (Fig. 17-5).

Prognosis

As with other cancers, the extent of spread is an important prognostic factor. Stage I disease involves only the skin. Stage II disease involves first-order lymph nodes or tissue sites between the primary tumor and first-order nodes. Stage III disease involves the central nervous system (i.e., brain), bones, or visceral organs. Stage I disease carries a relatively good prognosis compared with the dismal outcome of stage III disease.

For individuals with stage I disease, tumor thickness is the single most important indicator of prognosis because a direct correlation exists between tumor thickness and survival. In melanoma, tumor thickness is inversely related to survival. The Breslow Thickness Scale defines primary melanomas that are less than 0.76 mm as local tumors. These tumors have greater than 90% cure rates after simple excision. Individuals with tumors 0.76 to 4.0 mm thick have a greater than 80% risk of having distant disease and a less than 50% chance of 5-year survival. A second tumor classification system, Clark's Levels of Tumor Invasion, provides an anatomic description of tumor invasion. The level of tumor invasion can be used for discussing prognosis and planning surgical management (Fig. 17-6).

Treatment

Management strategies are predicated on the extent of disease. Treatment of primary localized disease differs greatly from that of metastatic disease.

In primary discrete lesions, total excisional biopsy with 2 cm margins is performed. Most tissue defects are closed primarily without skin grafting. If primary biopsy specimens are found to have tumor-negative margins, then no further surgical treatment is required. Primary mucosal melanomas have poor outcomes because disease is usually extensive. Nail bed lesions require amputation at the distal interphalangeal (DIP) joint for finger primaries and the interphalangeal (IP) joint for thumb primaries.

In regional disease, the performance of elective regional lymph node dissection for nonpalpable nodes

Figure 17-6 The Clark and Breslow classification for melanoma. (Reproduced by permission from Lawrence PF. Essentials of general surgery. Baltimore: Williams & Wilkins, 1988:355.)

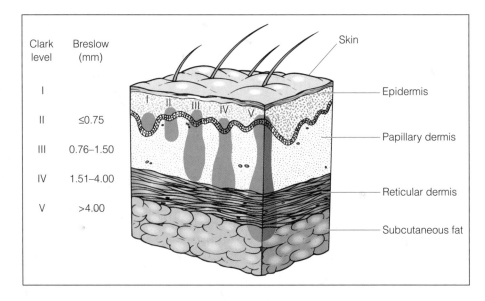

Clark level	Breslow (mm)
I	
II	≤0.75
III	0.76–1.50
IV	1.51–4.00
V	>4.00

Skin
Epidermis
Papillary dermis
Reticular dermis
Subcutaneous fat

remains controversial. Breslow's thickness scale and Clark's level of invasion are used to predict the chance of metastasis to first-order lymph nodes. Thin lesions limited to the epidermis have a low likelihood of lymph node metastasis, whereas thick lesions invading the subcutaneous fat have a high likelihood of systemic disease. Therefore, a surgeon tends to perform regional lymphadenectomy for thicker, higher level lesions versus thin, local lesions. Recently, lymphoscintigraphy has been used in the operating room to identify the "sentinel node" of the first-order lymph node basin into which the tumor initially drains. In lymphoscintigraphy, technetium and a sulfur colloid are circumferentialy injected around the primary lesion. The technetium then drains via lymphatics to the sentinel node, which is identified using a handheld scintigrapher. Once identified, the sentinel node is excised and evaluated microscopically for evidence of lymph node metastasis.

In metastatic disease, individuals with a single identifiable metastatic lesion may benefit from surgical resection. However, new metastatic lesions usually occur for which surgical intervention is unwarranted. Metastatic sites include skin, lung, brain, bone, liver, and the gastrointestinal tract. Treatment options include surgery, radiation, chemotherapy, and isolated limb perfusion.

Prevention

Professional and public education campaigns, combined with early diagnosis and appropriate surgical removal, increase survival for individuals diagnosed with melanoma.

Key Points
Melanoma

1. Is a potentially lethal skin cancer arising from melanocytes;

2. Is thought to be caused by ultraviolet light;

3. Arises mostly from pre-existing moles;

4. Has five signs: Asymmetric shape, irregular Border, mottled Color, large Diameter, and progressive Enlargement;

5. Has four types: superficial spreading, lentigo maligna, acral lentiginous, and nodular;

6. Prognosis for primary tumors is based on tumor thickness: tumors less than 0.76 mm have greater than 90% cure rates;

7. Primary tumors require excision with 2-cm margins;

8. Nail bed tumors require distal joint amputation;

9. Lymph node dissection confirms regional disease;

10. Sites of metastasis are lung, brain, bone, and the gastrointestinal tract.

▶ SQUAMOUS CELL CARCINOMA

Squamous cell carcinoma (SCC) is the second most common form of skin cancer after BCC. Tumors arise from the skin and the oral and anogenital mucosa. Multiple predisposing factors for developing SCC have been identified.

Pathogenesis

The predominant etiology of most SCC is chronic actinic damage that induces the malignant transformation of epidermal keratinocytes. A similar effect is seen with exposure to ionizing radiation (x-rays and gamma rays). In darkly pigmented individuals, however, most lesions arise from sites of chronic inflammation, such as osteomyelitis and chronic tropical ulcerations. Tumors also arise at mucocutaneous interfaces secondary to tobacco use or human papilloma virus (HPV) infection. Smokers typically present with ulcerating lip and gum or tongue lesions, whereas invasive cancers of the vulva and penis are seen with HPV infection. Anogenital SCC is linked to infection with HPV types 16, 18, 31, 33, and 35. Immunosuppressed or immunocompromised individuals, namely, transplant recipients on immunosuppressive medication or those with HIV/AIDS, have an increased incidence of squamous cell cancer and an elevated rate of metastasis. Rarely, tumors arise from old scars, usually sustained secondary to burn injury, which form so-called Marjolin's ulcers or burn scar tumors. As a rule, actinically induced cancers infrequently metastasize, whereas tumors arising from other mechanisms have a significantly higher rate of metastasis (Table 17-1).

TABLE 17-1

Predisposing Factors for Developing SCC

Sunlight exposure
Human papilloma virus infection
Immunosuppression (transplant recipients)
Immunocompromization (HIV infection)
Chronic ulcers
Ionizing radiation (x-rays, gamma rays)
Tobacco use
Scars (burn injury)

History

SCC presents as an indurated nodule or plaque, often with ulceration, which has slowly evolved over time. Most lesions are on sun-exposed areas such as the face, ears, and upper extremities.

Physical Examination

Whites exhibit pinkish lesions, whereas darker skinned individuals have hypo- or hyperpigmented lesions. Regional lymphadenopathy occurs in 35% of SCC arising in the lip and mouth. Aberrant keratinization is often seen in SCC, occasionally causing the growth of cutaneous horns. Therefore, the base of a cutaneous horn should always be examined for the presence of squamous cell cancer (Fig. 17-7).

Treatment

The preferred treatment is tumor removal by surgical excision. The remaining defect is closed either primarily for smaller lesions or by skin grafting or flap reconstruction for larger lesions. Cryosurgery or cautery/curettage can also be used for small tumors.

Prognosis

The overall cure rate for SCC is 90% after treatment. Tumors other than sun-induced SCC have a higher mortality rate due to the greater likelihood of metastasis.

Key Points

Squamous cell carcinoma

1. Is the second most common form of skin cancer;

2. Is predominantly caused by sunlight exposure;

3. May arise in oral and anogenital mucosa from tobacco use or HPV infection;

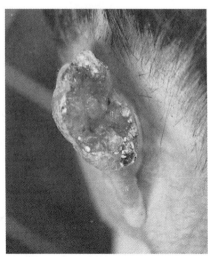

Figure 17-7 Squamous cell carcinoma.

4. Of the vulva and penis is associated with HPV type 16, 18, 31, 33 and 35 infection;

5. Has an increased incidence in immunosuppressed and immunocompromised individuals and exhibits an elevated risk of metastases;

6. May arise in old burn scars as Marjolin's ulcers;

7. May arise in sites of chronic inflammation, such as osteomyelitis and chronic ulcers;

8. Typically presents as an indurated nodule or plaque, often with ulceration;

9. Is treated by surgical excision;

10. Has an overall post-treatment cure rate of 90%.

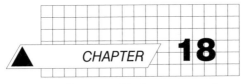

CHAPTER 18

Small Intestine

▶ ANATOMY AND PHYSIOLOGY

The small intestine comprises the duodenum, jejunum, and ileum and extends from the pylorus proximally to the cecum distally. Its main function is to digest and absorb nutrients. Absorption is achieved by the large surface area of the small intestine secondary to its long length and extensive mucosal projections of villi and microvilli. A broad-based mesentery suspends the small intestine from the posterior abdominal wall once the retroperitoneal duodenum emerges at the ligament of Treitz and becomes the jejunum. Arterial blood is supplied from branches of the superior mesenteric artery and venous drainage is via the superior mesenteric vein. The mucosa has sequential circular folds called plicae circulares. The plicae circulares are more numerous in the proximal bowel than distal bowel. The mucosal villi and microvilli create the surface through which carbohydrates, fats, proteins, and electrolytes are absorbed (Figs. 18-1 and 18-2).

▶ SMALL BOWEL OBSTRUCTION

Although the etiology of small bowel obstruction (SBO) is varied, the presentation of this disorder is usually quite consistent because if a common mechanism. Obstruction of the small bowel lumen causes progressive proximal accumulation of intraluminal fluids and gas. Peristalsis continues to transport swallowed air and secreted intestinal fluid through the bowel proximal to the obstruction, resulting in small bowel dilation and eventual abdominal distention. Depending on the location of the obstruction, vomiting will occur early in proximal obstruction and later in more distal blockage. Crampy abdominal pain initially occurs as active proximal peristalsis exacerbates bowel dilation. However, with progressive bowel wall edema and luminal dilation, peristaltic activity decreases and abdominal pain lessens. At presentation, patients exhibit abdominal distention and complain of mild diffuse abdominal pain (Fig. 18-3).

Etiology

The first and second most common causes of SBO are adhesions and hernias (Table 18-1). Most adhesions are caused by postoperative internal scar formation. Discovering the actual mechanism of obstruction is also important because it relates to the possibility of vascular compromise and bowel ischemia. For example, a closed-loop obstruction caused by volvulus with torsion is at high risk for vascular compromise. This is often seen when a loop of small bowel twists around an adhesion.

A second mechanism causing bowel ischemia is incarceration in a fixed space. Incarceration and subsequent strangulation impedes venous return, causing edema and eventual bowel infarction. Other mechanisms of obstruction that rarely compromise vascular flow are obturation of the bowel lumen by a gallstone or bezoar and intussusception caused by an intramural or mucosal lesion as the leading edge.

History

Patients usually present with complaints of intermittent crampy abdominal pain, abdominal distention, obstipation, nausea, and vomiting. Vomiting of feculent material usually occurs later in the course of obstruction. Constant localizable pain or pain out of proportion to physical findings may indicate ischemic bowel.

Physical Examination

A distended abdomen with diffuse midabdominal tenderness to palpation is usually found on physical examination. There are typically no signs of peritonitis. If constant localized tenderness is apparent, ischemia and gangrene must be suspected. An essential aspect of the examination is to check for abdominal wall hernias, especially in postsurgical patients. Elevation in temperature should not be present in uncomplicated cases. Tachycardia may be present from hypovolemia secondary to persistent vomiting or from toxemia caused by intestinal gangrene.

Diagnostic Evaluation

Plain upright radiographs classically demonstrate distended loops of small bowel with multiple air-fluid interfaces. Occasionally, the radiograph will elucidate the etiology of the obstruction, the site of obstruction, and whether the obstruction is partial or complete. Free air indicates perforation, whereas biliary gas and an opacity near the ileocecal valve is diagnostic for gallstone ileus.

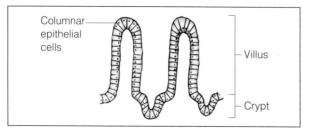

Figure 18-1 Electron micrograph of small intestinal villi.

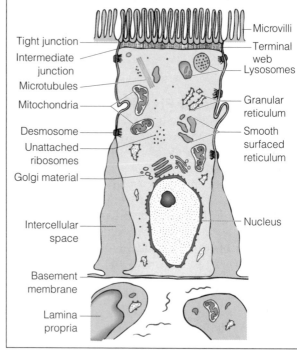

Figure 18-2 Diagram of a columnar epithelial intestinal absorptive cell.

Figure 18-3 Variable manifestations of SBO depend upon the level of blockage.

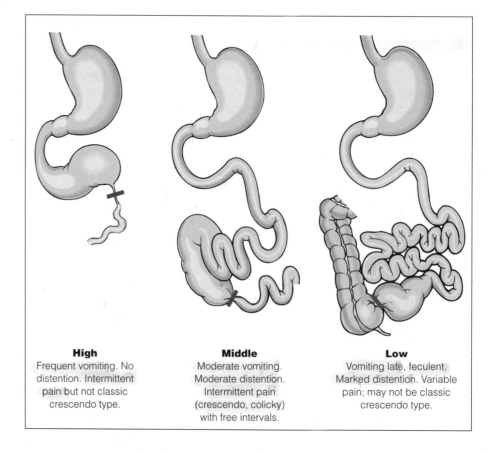

High
Frequent vomiting. No distention. Intermittent pain but not classic crescendo type.

Middle
Moderate vomiting. Moderate distention. Intermittent pain (crescendo, colicky) with free intervals.

Low
Vomiting late, feculent. Marked distention. Variable pain; may not be classic crescendo type.

TABLE 18-1
Causes of Small Bowel Obstruction

Adhesions
Hernias—abdominal wall, internal
Neoplasms—primary, metastatic
Obturation/strictures—ischemia, radiation, Crohn's, gallstone, bezoar
Intussusception
Meckel's diverticulum
Volvulus
Superior mesenteric artery syndrome
Intramural hematoma

Treatment

Initial treatment consists of nasogastric decompression to relieve proximal gastrointestinal distention and associated nausea and vomiting. Fluid resuscitation follows as patients are usually intravascularly depleted from persistent vomiting.

The decision to operate is based on the nature of the obstruction and the patient's condition. If ischemia or perforation is suspected, immediate operation is necessary. Otherwise, patients can be observed with serial physical examinations and radiographs. If the patient worsens or fails to improve with supportive therapy, then operative intervention is indicated.

Key Points
Small bowel

1. Obstructions are commonly caused by adhesions and hernias;

2. Patients complain of progressive abdominal distention, diffuse abdominal pain, nausea, and vomiting;

3. Infarction occurs with closed loop obstruction and with incarceration and strangulation; patients with peritonitis require surgery;

4. Many patients are successfully managed with supportive therapy alone;

5. Distended small bowel loops with multiple air-fluid interfaces are seen on x-ray in SBO. Biliary gas and a right lower quadrant opacity indicates gallstone ileus.

▶ CROHN'S DISEASE

Crohn's disease is a transmural inflammatory disease that may affect any part of the gastrointestinal tract, from the mouth to the anus. Ileal involvement is most common. The disease is characterized by "skip lesions" that involve discontinuous segments of abnormal mucosa. Granulomata are usually seen microscopically, but not always. Areas of inflammation are often associated with fibrotic strictures, enterocutaneous fistulas, and intra-abdominal abscesses, all of which generally require surgical intervention.

Epidemiology

Crohn's disease occurs throughout the world, although the actual incidence exhibits a geographic and ethnic variability. The incidence in the United States is about 10 times that of Japan. Ashkenazi Jews have a far higher incidence of disease than African-Americans.

Etiology

The etiology of Crohn's disease remains unknown. Because of the presence of granulomata, mycobacterial infection has been postulated as the causative agent. Recent investigations with *Mycobacterium paratuberculosis* have proven inconclusive. An immunologic basis for the disease has also been advanced; however, although humoral and cellular immune responses are involved in disease pathogenesis, no specific immunologic disturbance has been identified.

Pathology

The small intestine is affected in at least 70% of all patients with Crohn's disease. The ileum is typically diseased, with frequent right colon involvement. On gross inspection, the serosal surface of the bowel is hypervascular and the mesentery characteristically shows signs of "creeping fat." The bowel walls are edematous and fibrotic. The mucosa has a cobblestone appearance with varying degrees of associated mucosal ulceration. Histologically, a chronic lymphocytic infiltrate in an inflamed mucosa and submucosa is seen. Fissure ulcers penetrate deep into the mucosa and are often associated with granulomata and multinucleated giant cells. Granulomata are seen more frequently in distal tissues, which explains why granulomata are seen more often in colonic disease than in ileal disease.

History

Patients with Crohn's disease of the small bowel present complaining of diarrhea, abdominal pain, anorexia, nausea, and weight loss. The diarrhea is usually loose and watery without frank blood. Dull abdominal pain is usually in the right iliac fossa or periumbilical region. Children often present with symptoms of malaise and have noticeable growth failure. Strictures may cause partial SBO, resulting in bacterial overgrowth and subsequent steatorrhea, flatus, and bloating.

Physical Examination

Patients may appear to be either generally healthy or else they may have significant cachexia. Abdominal examination may reveal right iliac fossa tenderness. In acutely ill patients, a palpable abdominal mass may be present, indicating abscess formation. Enterocutaneous fistulae may be present. Oral examination may reveal evidence of mucosal ulceration, whereas perianal inspection may show skin tags, fissures, or fistulae. Extraintestinal manifestations include erythema nodosum, pyoderma gangrenosum, ankylosing spondylitis, and uveitis.

Diagnostic Evaluation

Blood studies often show a mild iron deficiency anemia and a depressed albumin level. If hypoalbuminemia is severe, then peripheral edema may be present.

Small intestine Crohn's disease is diagnosed by barium contrast enteroclysis. This small intestine enema technique provides better mucosal definition than standard small bowel follow-through studies. Aphthoid ulcers, strictures, fissures, bowel wall thickening, and fistulae are illustrated with this technique. Fistulograms are helpful to define existing fistula tracks, and CT can localize abscesses. Once radiographic evidence of disease is found, colonoscopy should be performed to evaluate the colonic mucosa and to obtain biopsies of the terminal ileum.

DDx

Acute appendicitis, *Yersinia* infection, lymphoma, intestinal tuberculosis, Behçet's disease.

Complications

Crohn's disease carries a high morbidity and low mortality. Small bowel strictures secondary to inflammation and fibrosis are common complications that present as obstruction. Fistulae from small bowel to adjacent loops of small bowel, large bowel, bladder, vagina, or skin also occur. Ileal Crohn's disease can result in gallstone formation because of the interruption of the enterohepatic circulation of bile salts. Kidney stones may also form because of hyperoxaluria. Normally, calcium and oxalate bind in the intestine and are excreted in the feces. With ileal Crohn's disease, steatorrhea causes ingested fat to bind intraluminal calcium, thus allowing free oxalate to be absorbed. Finally, adenocarcinoma is a rare complication that usually arises in the ileum.

Treatment

Mild disease can be controlled with a 4- to 6-week course of sulfasalazine or mesalazine. Alternatively,

TABLE 18-2

Indications for Surgery in Crohn's Disease

Stenosis with obstructive symptoms
Fistulae
Abscess
Perforation
Bleeding

oral corticosteroids may be used with equivalent results. Metronidazole may also be useful. Patients with bile salt-induced diarrhea after ileal resection may benefit from cholestyramine.

Severe disease is treated with hospitalization, bowel rest, hydration, intravenous nutrition, steroids, and metronidazole. Patients with chronic active disease may benefit from a course of 6-mercaptopurine.

Surgery in Crohn's disease should only be performed for complications of the disease (Table 18-2). Surgery should be conservative and address only the presenting indication, using gentle surgical technique. Resections should be avoided because overly aggressive intervention can produce surgically induced short bowel syndrome and malnutrition. Some common surgical problems encountered in Crohn's disease and their treatments include ileocolic disease, which is managed by conservative ileocecal resection to grossly normal margins (Fig. 18-4); stricture, which is managed by stricturoplasty that entails incising the antimesenteric border of the stricture along the intestinal long axis and then closing the enterotomy transversely (Fig. 18-5); and abscess/fistula, which is managed by open or percutaneous drainage of the abscess and resection of the small bowel segment responsible for initiating the fistula with primary anastomosis (Fig. 18-6).

Key Points

1. Crohn's disease is a transmural inflammatory process that effects any part of the gastrointestinal tract from the mouth to the anus.

2. The ileum is most commonly involved. Discontinuous mucosal "skip lesions" are seen macroscopically, with associated granulomata seen microscopically.

3. It has extraintestinal manifestations that include erythema nodosum, pyoderma gangrenosum, and uveitis.

4. Ileal disease may cause gallstones and kidney stones by the interruption of the enterohepatic circulation of bile salts and by increased gastrointestinal oxalate absorption.

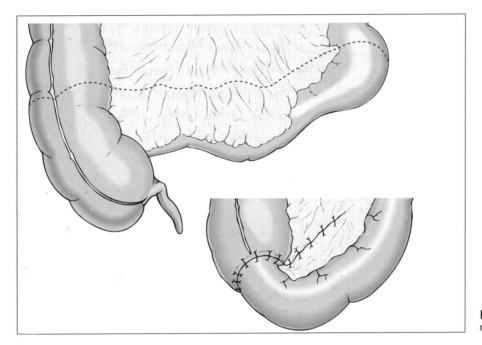

Figure 18-4 Ileocecal resection for Crohn's disease.

Figure 18-5 Stricturoplasty of a localized stricture with transverse closure.

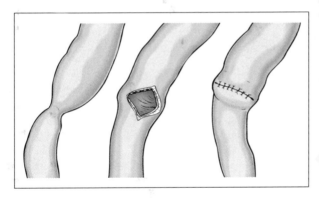

Figure 18-6 Fistula resection with end-to-end anastomosis.

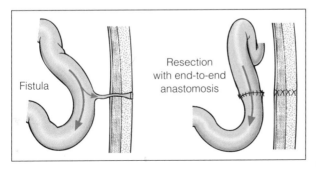

▶ MECKEL'S DIVERTICULUM

This most common congenital anomaly of the small intestine is an antimesenteric remnant arising from a failure of vitelline duct obliteration during embryonic development. Meckel's diverticula are true diverticula containing all three intestinal muscle layers. Diverticula are usually less than 12 cm in length and are found within 100 cm of the ileocecal valve.

Associated abnormalities of the vitelline duct depend on the degree of duct obliteration that occurs during development. Complete ductal obliteration leaves a thin fibrous band connecting ileum to umbilicus, whereas complete duct persistence results in a patent ileoumbilical fistula. Partial obstruction results in cyst or blind sinus formation. Heterotopic tissue (gastric, pancreatic) is found in 30% to 50% of diverticula (Fig. 18-7).

Complications

Bleeding within the diverticulum may occur from peptic ulceration arising from heterotopic gastric mucosa. In infants, Meckel's diverticulum is the most common cause of major lower gastrointestinal bleeding.

Bowel obstruction may result from one of two mechanisms: intussusception can occur when an inverted diverticulum functions as a lead point and small

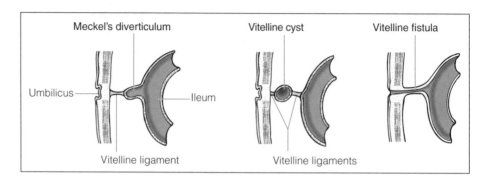

Figure 18-7 Vitelline duct remnants.

bowel volvulus can occur around a fixed obliterated vitelline duct extending from the ileum to the umbilicus.

Diagnostic Evaluation

For Meckel's diverticula containing heterotopic gastric mucosa, the Tc-99 scan is helpful for diagnosis. Pertechnetate anions are taken up by ectopic gastric parietal cells and indicate diverticulum location. Diverticula not containing heterotopic gastric tissue can occasionally be visualized using standard barium contrast studies.

Treatment

Definitive treatment for the complications of Meckel's diverticulum is by surgical resection.

Key Points

Meckel's diverticulum

1. Is the most common congenital abnormality of the small intestine and arises from a failure of vitelline duct obliteration;

2. Is a true diverticulum and may contain heterotopic gastric and pancreatic tissue;

3. May develop peptic ulceration, the most common cause of major lower gastrointestinal bleeding in infants.

▶ SMALL BOWEL TUMORS

Tumors of the small bowel are rare, accounting for 1% to 5% of all gastrointestinal tumors. Most tumors are benign. Common benign neoplasms of the small bowel include tubular and villous adenomas, lipomas, leiomyomas, and hemangiomas. Telangiectasias of Osler-Rendu-Weber syndrome, neurofibromas of neurofibromatosis, hamartomatous polyps of Peutz-Jeghers syndrome and heterotopic tissue as in Meckel's diverticulum are also found. Possible explanations for this lack of malignancy include short exposure to ingested carcinogens secondary to rapid transit time, low bacterial counts resulting in fewer endogenously produced carcinogens, and the intraluminal secretion of immunoglobulin A by small bowel mucosa.

Benign lesions are generally asymptomatic and are incidental findings. Of symptomatic lesions, obstruction is the most common presentation, followed by hemorrhage. In the workup of gastrointestinal bleeding, however, unless other evidence exists, small bowel lesions should be low on the list of differential diagnoses because greater than 90% of bleeding lesions occur between the esophagus and distal duodenum and from between the ileocecal valve and anus. Small bowel lesions should be suspected if careful skin examination reveals café-au-lait spots (neurofibromatosis), telangiectasia (Osler-Rendu-Weber syndrome), or mucocutaneous pigmentation (Peutz-Jeghers syndrome).

Diagnostic Evaluation

Visual endoscopic identification of small bowel tumors is generally possible for those lesions of the proximal duodenum and terminal ileum. The remainder of the small bowel requires examination by barium contrast studies. For larger lesions, CT may be helpful.

In situations involving active hemorrhage, Tc-99 sulfur colloid or Tc-99-labeled red blood cell studies may show the bleeding site. However, a bleeding rate of 1 cc/minute is required for accurate localization.

When available diagnostic modalities are insufficient, exploratory laparotomy may be necessary. In addition to external inspection at laparotomy, operative endoscopy may be used for intraluminal evaluation.

Key Points

Small bowel tumors

1. Are rare and generally benign;

2. Most commonly present as small bowel obstruction;

3. Are mostly benign adenomas, lipomas, leiomyomas, and hemangiomas;

4. Occur frequently in neurofibromatosis, Osler-Rendu-Weber, and Peutz-Jeghers syndromes.

▶ CARCINOID

Carcinoid tumors are the most common endocrine tumors of the gastrointestinal tract, constituting over half of all such lesions. They account for up to 30% of all small bowel tumors. Carcinoid tumors arise from neuroendocrine enterochromaffin cells. Hence, tumors can secrete serotonin and other humoral substances such as histamine, dopamine, tachykinins, peptides, and prostaglandins. The metabolite of serotonin, 5-hydroxyindoleacetic acid (5-HIAA), is excreted in the urine and is easily detected. Carcinoid tumor cells also have APUD (amine precursor uptake and decarboxylation) characteristics. Namely, they are cells with cytoplasm high in Amine content, cells capable of amine Precursor Uptake, and cells capable of Decarboxylating precursors to form amines or peptides.

All carcinoids are considered malignant due to their potential for invasion and metastasis. Patients with metastatic disease manifest the carcinoid syndrome that consists of the systemic effects (flushing, diarrhea, sweating, and wheezing) of secreted vasoactive substances. Presence of the carcinoid syndrome indicates hepatic metastasis, because systemic effects occur when venous drainage from a tumor escapes hepatic metabolism of vasoactive substances.

About 85% of carcinoid tumors are found in the intestine and about 50% are found in the appendix, making it the most common site of occurrence, followed by the ileum, jejunum, rectum, and duodenum. Other sites of disease include the lungs and occasionally the pancreas and biliary tract. Appendiceal carcinoids rarely metastasize, whereas lesions of the ileum have the highest association with carcinoid syndrome. Jejunoileal carcinoids are frequently multicentric.

History

The clinical presentation of patients with carcinoid tumors will differ depending on tumor location. Primary tumors may present as SBO because tumors can incite an intense local fibrosis of the bowel that causes angulation and kinking of the involved segment. As noted, metastatic disease with hepatic spread is manifested by the carcinoid syndrome. Occult primary lesions do not cause systemic effects because 5-hydroxytryptamine (seratonin) is metabolized by the liver. Other presenting symptoms can include abdominal pain, upper intestinal or rectal bleeding, intussusception, weight loss, or a palpable abdominal mass.

Diagnostic Evaluation

Laboratory studies should include plasma and urine analysis to evaluate for elevated levels of plasma serotonin and urinary 5-HIAA.

Barium contrast studies are also useful for diagnosing carcinoid tumors. Barium enemas can demonstrate lesions of the rectum and large bowel, whereas small bowel enteroclysis may show a discrete lesion or a stricture secondary to fibrosis. Because primary tumors are usually small, CT is usually only helpful for detecting hepatic metastases. Colonoscopy can visualize tumors from the terminal ileum to the rectum.

Treatment

Surgical resection of the primary tumor is always undertaken, even in cases of metastatic disease. If the tumor is left in situ, bowel obstruction and intussusception will ultimately result. At laparotomy, adequate bowel and mesenteric margins must be obtained, as with any cancer operation. Depending on tumor size and the degree of spread, lesions can be treated with simple local excision for small primaries to wide en bloc resection for metastatic disease.

Patients suffering from carcinoid syndrome can achieve symptomatic relief with daily subcutaneous injections of the somatostatin analogue, octreotide. Parenthetically, induction with general anesthesia may provoke a life-threatening carcinoid crisis characterized by hypotension, flushing, tachycardia, and arrhythmias. Intravenous somatostatin or octreotide will rapidly reverse the crisis.

Prognosis

Survival for patients with carcinoid tumors is directly related to the size of the primary tumor and to the presence of metastasis. For noninvasive lesions of the appendix and rectum less than 2 cm in size, the 5-year survival rate nears 100%. As the tumor size increases, the survival rate decreases. The presence of muscle wall invasion and positive lymph nodes are poor prognostic signs. Patients with hepatic metastases have an average survival of approximately 3 years. Liver lesions are usually multiple and therefore unresectable. Palliation is achieved with octreotide therapy or chemoembolization.

Key Points

Carcinoid tumors

1. Are the most common endocrine tumors of the gastrointestinal tract;

2. Most commonly occur in the appendix;

3. Are all considered malignant because of their potential for invasion and metastasis;

4. Secrete serotonin, which is broken down in the liver to the metabolite 5-HIAA that is excreted in the urine.

Carcinoid syndrome

1. Is manifested as flushing, diarrhea, sweating, and wheezing, and is caused by the systemic effects of secreted vasoactive substances;

2. Invariably indicates hepatic metastases because vasoactive substances have escaped hepatic metabolism;

3. Is treated by octreotide therapy and chemoembolization to provide symptomatic relief.

CHAPTER 19

Stomach and Duodenum

*7*he stomach and duodenum are discussed as a single unit because they are anatomically contiguous structures, share an inter-related physiology, and suffer similar disease processes. Peptic ulceration is the most common inflammatory disorder of the gastrointestinal tract and is responsible for significant disability. The stomach and duodenum are principally affected by peptic ulceration.

▶ ANATOMY

The stomach is divided into the fundus, body, and antrum (Fig. 19-1). The fundus is the superior dome of the stomach, the body extends from the fundus to the angle of the stomach (incisura angularis) located on the lesser curvature, and the antrum extends from the body to the pylorus. Hydrochloric acid-secreting parietal cells are found in the fundus, pepsinogen-secreting chief cells are found in the proximal stomach, and gastrin-secreting G cells are found in the antrum.

Six arterial sources supply blood to the stomach: the left and right gastric arteries to the lesser curvature, the left and right gastroepiploic arteries to the greater curvature, the short gastric arteries branching from the splenic artery to supply the fundus, and the gastroduodenal artery branches to the pylorus. The vagus nerve supplies parasympathetic innervation via the anterior left and posterior right trunks. These nerves stimulate gastric motility and the secretion of pepsinogen and hydrochloric acid (Fig. 19-2).

The duodenum is divided into four portions (Fig. 19-3). The first portion begins at the pylorus and includes the duodenal bulb. The ampulla of Vater, through which the common bile duct and pancreatic duct drain, is located in the medial wall of the descending second portion of the duodenum. The transverse third portion is traversed anteriorly by the superior mesenteric vessels. The ascending fourth portion terminates at the ligament of Treitz, which defines the duodenal-jejunal junction. The arterial supply to the duodenum is via the superior pancreaticoduodenal artery, which arises from the gastroduodenal artery, and by the inferior pancreaticoduodenal artery, which arises from the superior mesenteric artery.

▶ GASTRIC AND DUODENAL ULCERATION

Pathogenesis

The etiology of benign peptic gastric and duodenal ulceration involves a compromised mucosal surface undergoing acid-peptic digestion. Substances that alter mucosal defenses include nonsteroidal anti-inflammatory drugs (NSAIDs), alcohol, and tobacco use. Alcohol directly attacks the mucosa, NSAIDs alter prostaglandin synthesis, and smoking restricts mucosal vascular perfusion. Recent evidence suggests that infestation with the organism *Helicobacter pylori* plays an important role in the pathogenesis of gastric and duodenal ulceration. Acid hypersecretion has been documented in at least 50% of patients with duodenal ulceration. Acid hypersecretion has not been documented in patients with gastric ulceration; in fact, most patients with gastric ulcers secrete less than average levels of acid but still enough to maintain a luminal pH of about 3.

History

Patients typically present complaining of epigastric pain relieved by food or antacids. Sensations of fullness and mild nausea are common, but vomiting is rare unless pyloric obstruction is present secondary to scarring. Physical examination is often benign except for occasional epigastric tenderness.

Diagnostic Evaluation

The radiographic evaluation of peptic ulcers entails barium studies that reveal evidence of crater deformities at areas of ulceration (Figs. 19-4 and 19-5).

Definitive diagnosis is made by direct visualization of the ulcer using endoscopy. For nonhealing gastric ulcers refractory to medical therapy, it is extremely important that biopsy of the ulcer be performed to rule out gastric carcinoma.

Treatment

Medical treatment is similar for both gastric and duodenal ulceration. The goals of medical therapy are to decrease production or neutralize stomach acid and to enhance mucosal protection against acid attack. Medications include antacids ($CaCO_3$), H_2-blockers (cimetidine,

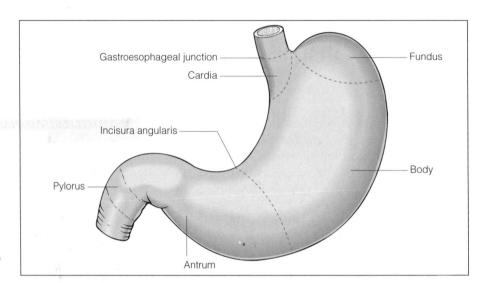

Figure 19-1 Anatomy of the stomach.

Figure 19-2 Blood supply and parasympathetic innervation of the stomach and duodenum.

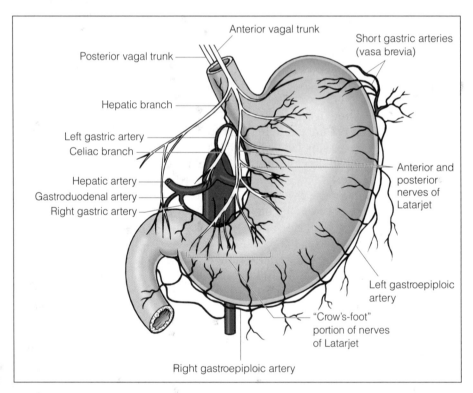

ranitidine), mucosal coating agents (sucralfate), prostaglandins (misoprostol), and proton-pump inhibitors (omeprazole). Treatment of *H. pylori* with oral antibiotics is associated with a 90% eradication rate. Treatment regimens may consist of tetracycline/metronidazole/bismuth subsalicylate, amoxicillin/metronidazole/ranitidine, or other combinations.

Surgical treatment for gastric ulceration in the acute setting is indicated by either perforation or massive bleeding. Indications for elective operation are a nonhealing ulcer after medical therapy and gastric outlet obstruction manifested by repeated vomiting, hyponatremia, and hypochloremia. The operation chosen must address the indication for which the procedure

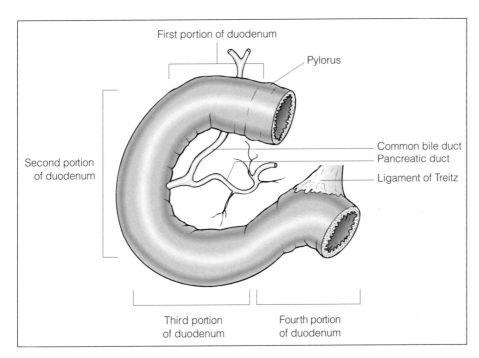

First portion of duodenum

Pylorus

Second portion of duodenum

Common bile duct
Pancreatic duct
Ligament of Treitz

Third portion of duodenum

Fourth portion of duodenum

Figure 19-3 Anatomy of the duodenum.

Figure 19-4 Gastric ulcer of the lesser curve.

Figure 19-5 Postbulbar duodenal ulcer.

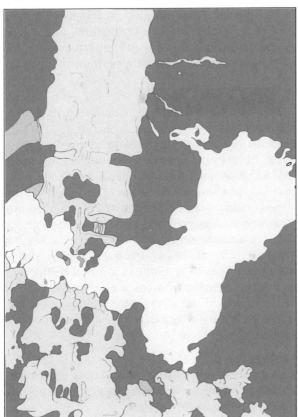

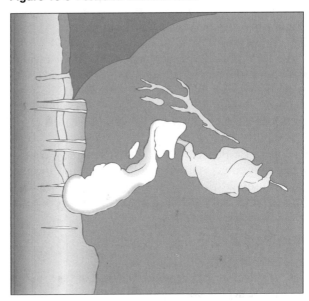

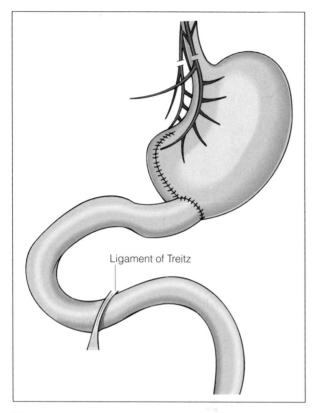

Figure 19-6 Vagotomy and Billroth I anastomosis.

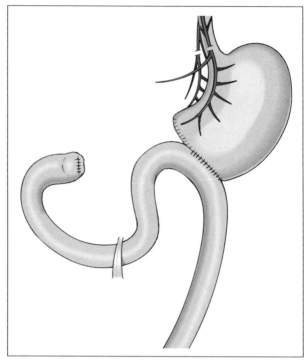

Figure 19-7 Vagotomy and Billroth II anastomosis.

is performed, perform excisional biopsy of the ulcer to rule out neoplasia, and permanently reduce acid secretion by removal of the entire antrum. In most instances, vagotomy and distal gastrectomy with Billroth I or II anastomosis will fulfill these criteria (Figs. 19-6 and 19-7).

Because denervation of the stomach by truncal vagotomy alters normal patterns of gastric motility and causes gastric atony, surgical drainage procedures are required after gastric denervation to ensure satisfactory gastric emptying.

Key Points
Peptic ulceration

1. Involves a compromised mucosal surface undergoing acid-peptic digestion;

2. Can be caused by NSAIDs, alcohol, and tobacco use, which alter mucosal defenses;

3. Has a pathogenesis linked to *H. pylori* infestation;

4. Is treated by decreasing stomach acidity and enhancing mucosal protection; *H. pylori* is eradicated with oral antibiotic therapy;

5. Is treated surgically for perforation, massive bleeding, gastric outlet obstruction, and a non-healing ulcer; vagotomy and antrectomy with Billroth anastomosis is usually performed.

▶ STRESS GASTRITIS AND ULCERATION
Pathogenesis
Critically ill patients subjected to severe physiologic stress, often in the intensive care unit setting, are at risk for developing gastroduodenal mucosal erosion that can progress to ulceration. The commonly accepted etiology of stress gastritis and ulceration is mucosal ischemia induced by an episode of hypotension from hemorrhage, sepsis, hypovolemia, or cardiac dysfunction. Ischemia disrupts cellular mechanisms of mucosal protection, resulting in mucosal acidification and superficial erosion. Areas of erosion may coalesce and form superficial ulcers. Stress ulcers are always found in the fundus and may be seen throughout the stomach and proximal duodenum.

History
Patients are usually critically ill and have a recent history of hypotension. Massive upper gastrointestinal bleeding is the usual finding.

Diagnostic Evaluation

Sites of hemorrhage can be identified by endoscopy.

Treatment

Endoscopy can often control bleeding by either electrocoagulation or photocoagulation. Persistent or recurrent bleeding unresponsive to endoscopic techniques requires surgical intervention. Depending on the circumstances, operations for control of bleeding stress gastritis or ulcer require oversewing of the bleeding vessel. Usually, vagotomy is also performed to reduce acid secretion. In many cases, bleeding cannot be controlled by suture ligation so partial or total gastrectomy is performed.

Prevention

Prevention of stress ulceration involves maintaining blood pressure, tissue perfusion, and acid-base stability and by decreasing acid production while bolstering mucosal protection. The incidence of life-threatening hemorrhagic gastritis has decreased as intravenous H_2-blocker therapy and oral cytoprotectants have been introduced to the intensive care setting.

Key Points

Stress gastritis and ulceration

1. Are secondary to mucosal ischemia caused by an episode of hypotension;
2. Areas of erosion coalesce to form ulceration;
3. May be treated by endoscopic coagulation or partial gastrectomy, if required;
4. Anti-ulcer prophylaxis and the maintenance of mucosal perfusion prevent stress ulceration.

▶ CUSHING'S ULCER

Distinct from stress gastritis, Cushing's ulcers are seen in patients with intracranial pathology (e.g., tumors, head injury). Ulcers are single and deep and may involve the esophagus, stomach, and duodenum. Because of the depth of ulceration, perforation is a common complication. Neuronally mediated acid hypersecretion is thought to be the main etiology of Cushing's ulcer.

Key Point

Cushing's ulcer

1. Occurs in patients with intracranial pathology, most probably secondary to neuronally mediated acid hypersecretion.

▶ ZOLLINGER-ELLISON SYNDROME AND GASTRINOMAS

Pathogenesis

Zollinger-Ellison syndrome occurs in a patient with severe peptic ulceration, and evidence of a gastrinoma (non-B-cell pancreatic tumor). Peptic ulceration results from the production of large volumes of highly acidic gastric secretions because of elevated serum gastrin levels. Ninety percent of gastrinomas are found in the "gastrinoma triangle" defined by the junction of the cystic duct and the common bile duct, the junction of the second and third portions of the duodenum, and the junction of the neck and body of the pancreas.

History

Gastrin-secreting tumors produce a clinical picture of epigastric pain, weight loss, vomiting, and severe diarrhea.

Diagnostic Evaluation

Diagnosis is confirmed by the secretin stimulation test where the injection of intravenous secretin elevates serum gastrin levels to at least 200 pg/mL. Once diagnosed, tumor localization is performed by either MRI, abdominal ultrasound, CT, selective abdominal angiography, or selective venous sampling.

Treatment

Acid hypersecretion can be controlled medically with H_2-blockade and proton pump inhibition. Somatostatin analogues (octreotide) have been found effective in decreasing tumor secretion of gastrin and in controlling the growth of tumor metastases.

Gastrinoma is a curable disease despite the malignant nature of most tumors. Complete resection of tumors results in a near 100% 10-year survival rate. Incomplete resection or unresectability carries a less than 50% 10-year survival rate. When simple excision or enucleation for cure is not feasible, an attempt is made to prolong survival by debulking and performing lymph node dissection to reduce tumor burden and acid hypersecretion.

Key Points

Gastrinomas

1. Cause Zollinger-Ellison syndrome, which is seen in patients with severe peptic ulceration, elevated serum gastrin levels, and evidence of a tumor within the "gastrinoma triangle";
2. Diagnosis is confirmed by the secretin stimulation test;

3. Medical treatment includes H_2-blockade, proton pump inhibition, and somastatin analogues;

4. Complete surgical resection can be curative.

▶ STOMACH CANCER

Despite the decreasing incidence of gastric carcinoma in Western populations over the past decades, patient survival has not improved. In the United States, less than 10% of patients with stomach cancer survive 5 years. Illustrative of geographic variation, stomach cancer is endemic in Japan. Because of the high incidence of disease, mass screening programs are able to detect early stage lesions, which accounts for a 50% overall survival rate at 5 years.

Risk Factors

Environmental and dietary factors are thought to influence the development of gastric cancer. Smoked fish and meats contain benzopyrene, a probable carcinogen to gastric mucosa. Nitrosamines are known carcinogens that are formed by the conversion of dietary nitrogen to nitrosamines in the gastrointestinal tract by bacterial metabolism. Atrophic gastritis, as seen in patients with hypogammaglobulinemia and pernicious anemia, is considered to be a premalignant condition for developing gastric cancer because high gastric pH encourages bacterial growth. Chronic atrophic gastritis results in achlorhydria, and 75% of patients with gastric cancer are achlorhydric.

Pathology

Most tumors are adenocarcinomas and spread is via lymphatics, venous drainage, and direct extension. Most tumors are located in the antral prepyloric region.

Gastric tumors can be typed according to gross appearance. Polypoid fungating nodular tumors are usually well differentiated and carry a relatively good prognosis after surgery. Ulcerating or penetrating tumors are the most common and are often mistaken for benign peptic ulcers because of their sessile nature. Superficial spreading lesions diffusely infiltrate through mucosa and submucosa and have a poor prognosis because most are metastatic at the time of diagnosis.

The pathologic staging of gastric cancer is based on depth of tumor invasion and lymph node status. The pathologic stage of a specific tumor correlates closely with survival (Fig. 19-8).

History

Patients with gastric cancer usually give a history of vague and nonspecific symptoms. Upper abdominal discomfort, dyspepsia, early satiety, belching, weight loss, anorexia, nausea, vomiting, hematemesis, or melena are common. Definite symptoms do not occur until tumor growth causes luminal obstruction, until tumor infiltration causes gastric dysmotility, or erosion causes bleeding. By the time of diagnosis, tumors are usually unresectable. Later symptoms indicative of metastatic disease are abdominal distention due to ascites from hepatic or peritoneal metastases and dyspnea and pleural effusions from pulmonary metastases.

Physical Examination

Few findings are noted on physical examination except in advanced disease. A firm, nontender, mobile epigastric mass may be palpated, and hepatomegaly with ascites may be present. Other distant signs of metastatic disease include Virchow's supraclavicular sentinel node, Sister Mary Joseph's umbilical node, and Blumer's shelf on rectal examination.

Diagnostic Evaluation

Anemia is often found on routine blood studies. The anemia is usually hypochromic and microcytic secondary to iron deficiency. Stool is often positive for occult blood.

In recent years, upper endoscopy has replaced the barium contrast upper gastrointestinal study as the imaging modality of choice. Endoscopy allows direct visualization and biopsy of the tumor. At least four biopsies should be made of the lesion. With 10 biopsies, the diagnostic accuracy approaches 100%. In Japan, the double contrast air/barium study is used extensively for screening. Once diagnosis is made, CT is performed to evaluate local extension and to look for evidence of ascites or metastatic disease.

Treatment

The theory behind curative resection involves en bloc primary tumor resection with wide disease-free margins and disease-free lymph nodes. Tumors are located either in the proximal, middle, or distal stomach. The type of operation performed for cure depends on tumor location.

Distal lesions located in the antral or prepyloric area are treated with Billroth II or Roux-en-Y anastomosis. The Billroth I procedure, used widely for benign peptic ulcer disease, is contraindicated when operating for gastric cancer (Fig. 19-9).

Midgastric lesions are treated with radical total gastrectomy with extensive lymph node dissection. The lesser and greater omentum are removed along with the spleen. If the body or tail of the pancreas are

Figure 19-8 Staging system for gastric carcinoma.

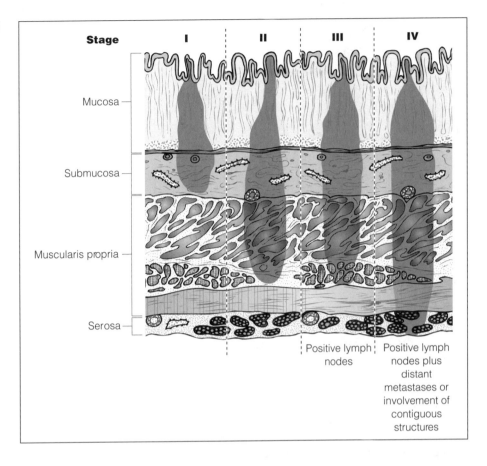

involved, distal pancreatectomy may be performed. Reconstruction is by Roux-en-Y anastomosis (Fig. 19-10).

Proximal lesions carry a poor prognosis and surgical intervention is usually palliative. Preoperative evaluation must include distal esophageal biopsies to determine whether there is esophageal involvement. For a simple proximal lesion, extended total gastrectomy with Roux-en-Y reconstruction is performed. If there is extension into the distal esophagus, then the esophagus is resected to the level of the azygos vein along with the cardia and lesser curvature. The remaining stomach tube is closed and the proximal aspect is anastomosed to the midesophagus through a right thoracotomy. If extensive esophageal involvement is discovered, then radical near-total gastrectomy and a near-complete esophagectomy are performed with continuity restored using a distal transverse colon and proximal left colon interpositon (Fig. 19-11).

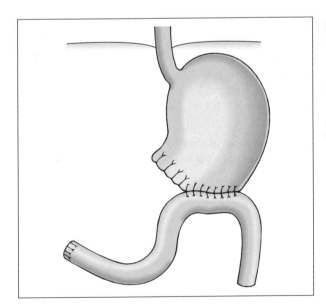

Figure 19-9 Billroth II reconstruction after antral gastric cancer resection.

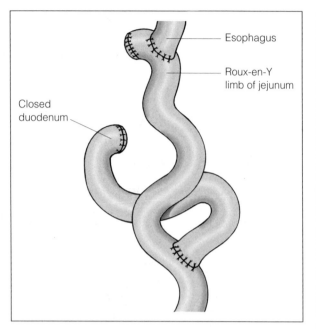

Figure 19-10 Roux-en-Y reconstruction after total gastrectomy.

Prognosis

The overall 5-year survival rate for gastric cancer in the United States is about 10%. Based on pathologic staging of tumors, the survival rate for stage I is 70%, stage II 30%, stage III 10%, and stage IV 0%.

Key Points

In stomach cancer,

1. Benzopyrene, nitrosamines, and atrophic gastritis are thought to influence the development of gastric cancer;

2. Most tumors are located in the antral region and are either polypoid nodular, ulcerating, or superficial spreading tumors on gross inspection;

3. The pathologic staging of gastric cancer is based on the depth of invasion and lymph node status;

4. Tumor stage correlates closely with survival;

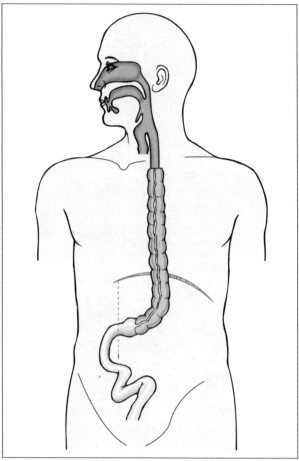

Figure 19-11 Colonic interposition after near-total esophagectomy and near-total gastrectomy.

5. Signs of metastatic disease include Virchow's node, Sister Mary Joseph's node, and Blumer's shelf;

6. The Billroth I anastomosis is contraindicated when operating for gastric cancer; en bloc resection with Billroth II or Roux-en-Y anastomoses is usually performed;

7. Esophageal involvement requires esophagectomy and gastrectomy with colonic interposition reconstruction.

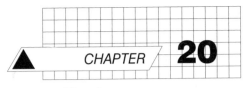

CHAPTER 20

Spleen

*T*he spleen is a purplish lymphatic organ located in the left upper abdominal quadrant. It contains the largest accumulation of lymphoid cells in the body and plays an important role in host defense, in addition to filtering the blood. Splenic lymphocytes are involved in antigen recognition and plasma cell production, whereas splenic endothelial macrophages extract bacteria and damaged red blood cells from the circulation by phagocytosis.

Surgical issues regarding the spleen are multiple and varied. Life-threatening hemorrhage from a lacerated spleen resulting from trauma is a common problem requiring swift surgical intervention. Certain disease states such as immune thrombocytopenic purpura (ITP) and the hemolytic anemias are often treated by splenectomy when medical management fails. Splenectomy may be necessary as part of another operation, such as distal pancreatectomy. Also, the traditional staging workup for Hodgkin's disease has involved removal of the spleen to determine extent of disease.

▶ ANATOMY

The spleen is embryologically derived from condensations of mesoderm in the dorsal mesogastrium of the developing gastrointestinal tract. In the mature abdomen, the spleen is found attached to the stomach by the gastrosplenic ligament and to the left kidney by the splenorenal ligament. Other supporting attachments include the splenocolic and splenophrenic ligaments (Fig. 20-1).

Accessory spleens are present in about 25% of patients. They are most often found in the splenic hilum and in the supporting splenic ligaments and greater omentum.

Arterial blood is mostly supplied via the splenic artery, which is one of three branches of the celiac axis (splenic, left gastric, common hepatic). At the hilum, the splenic artery divides into smaller branches that supply the several splenic segments. Additional arterial blood is supplied via the short gastric and left gastroepiploic vessels.

Venous drainage is from segmental veins that join at the splenic hilum to form the splenic vein. Running behind the upper edge of the pancreas, the splenic vein joins with the superior mesenteric vein to form the portal vein (Fig. 20-2).

Key Points

1. The spleen is a lymphatic organ that plays roles in antigen recognition and blood filtering.
2. Possible indications for splenectomy include hemorrhage, disease states, surgical resections, and rarely staging for Hodgkin's disease.
3. Accessory spleens occur in 25% of patients and are most commonly found in the splenic hilum.
4. Arterial blood is supplied via the splenic artery, the short gastric arteries, and branches of the left gastroepiploic artery.

▶ SPLENIC HEMORRHAGE

The most common cause of splenic hemorrhage is blunt abdominal trauma. Nonpenetrating injury may cause disruption of the splenic capsule or frank laceration of the splenic parenchyma. Displaced rib fractures of the left lower chest often cause splenic laceration.

Splenic hemorrhage may also be iatrogenic. Intraoperative damage to the spleen may occur during unrelated abdominal surgery that results in bleeding controlled only by splenectomy. Estimates are that 20% of splenectomies result from iatrogenic etiologies.

Infectious diseases (mononucleosis, malaria) may damage the spleen to the point where unnoticed blunt trauma can cause "spontaneous" splenic rupture and hemorrhage.

History

Patients typically present with a recent history of trauma, usually to the left upper abdomen or left flank.

Physical Examination

Depending on the degree of splenic injury and hemoperitoneum, a physical examination may reveal left upper quadrant abdominal tenderness, left lower rib fractures, abdominal distention, peritonitis, and hypovolemic shock.

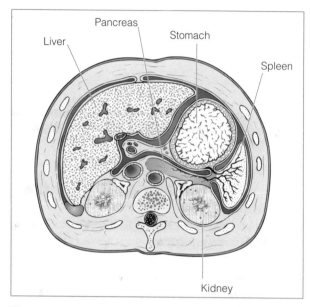

Figure 20-1 Normal anatomic relations of the spleen.

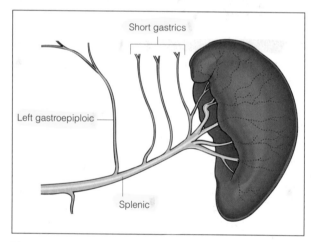

Figure 20-2 Arterial supply of the spleen.

Diagnostic Evaluation

Peritoneal lavage, abdominal ultrasound, or CT may be used to detect intraperitoneal blood. In hemodynamically stable patients, CT can demonstrate the degree of both splenic injury and hemoperitoneum.

Treatment

For patients with splenic injury who are hemodynamically stable and without evidence of ongoing hemorrhage, nonoperative management with close hemodynamic monitoring is becoming the accepted treatment of choice. In children, nonoperative management is widely applied due to the increased incidence of over-whelming postsplenectomy sepsis (OPSS) seen in the pediatric population. For patients with known or suspected splenic injury who are hemodynamically unstable, operative intervention is indicated for control of ongoing hemorrhage.

Once in the operating room, the decision to perform splenic repair (splenorrhaphy) versus splenectomy is based on the degree of injury to the parenchyma and blood supply of the organ. Relatively minor injuries such as a small capsular laceration with minor oozing may be repaired, whereas a fragmented spleen with involvement of the hilar vessels necessitates surgical removal.

Key Points

1. Hemorrhage secondary to trauma is the most common indication for splenectomy.

2. Nonoperative management or organ-sparing splenorrhaphy may be attempted because of the risk of OPSS, especially in children.

3. Hemodynamically stable patients may be managed nonoperatively.

► IMMUNE THROMBOCYTOPENIC PURPURA

ITP is an autoimmune hematologic disease where antiplatelet immunoglobulin IgG antibodies produced largely in the spleen are directed against a platelet associated antigen, resulting in platelet destruction by the reticuloendothelial system and subsequent thrombocytopenia. The disease is typically seen in young women who may present with complaints of menorrhagia, easy bruising, mucosal bleeding, and petechiae. Men may present with complaints of prolonged bleeding after shaving trauma.

Treatment

Initial therapy is with corticosteroids which improve platelet counts after 3 to 7 days of therapy. For prolonged active bleeding, platelet transfusions should be administered to achieve hemostasis.

Few patients enjoy complete and sustained remission with steroid treatment alone. Patients typically become refractory to medical treatment and thrombocytopenia recurs. Splenectomy is then indicated. After splenectomy, approximately 80% of patients develop normal platelet counts because the organ of both significant antiplatelet antibody production and platelet destruction is removed.

► HYPERSPLENISM

Hypersplenism describes a state of increased splenic function resulting in various hematologic abnormalities that may be normalized by splenectomy. Elevated splenic function causes a depression of the formed blood elements that leads to a compensatory hyperplasia of the bone marrow.

History

As in ITP, most patients are women who present with signs of anemia, recurrent infections, or easy bruising.

Physical Examination

Abdominal examination reveals splenomegaly.

Diagnostic Evaluation

Peripheral blood smear may reveal leukopenia, anemia, thrombocytopenia, or pancytopenia. Bone marrow biopsy shows pancellular hyperplasia.

Treatment

Splenectomy may produce hematologic improvement.

► HEMOLYTIC ANEMIAS

Hemolytic anemias are characterized by an elevated rate of red cell destruction from either a congenital or acquired etiology. Congenital hemolytic anemias result from basic defects of either the cell membrane (hereditary spherocytosis), hemoglobin synthesis (thalassemia), hemoglobin structure (sickle cell anemia), and cellular metabolism (G-6-PD deficiency). Acquired autoimmune hemolytic anemias result when antibodies are produced that are directed against the body's own red blood cells.

Diagnostic Evaluation

A positive direct Coombs' test demonstrates complexed antibodies on the red blood cell membrane. Warm-reactive antibodies are IgG and cold-reactive antibodies are IgM.

Treatment

The role of splenectomy in treating hemolytic anemias depends on the particular disease process. For example, red blood cell survival normalizes after splenectomy for hereditary spherocytosis, whereas operative intervention has no role in the treatment of anemia of G-6-PD deficiency that is secondary to a defect of metabolism, not cellular structure. Occasionally, splenectomy may be useful in selected patients with sickle cell anemia and thalassemia. Patients with autoimmune hemolytic anemias undergo initial steroid treatment and progress to splenectomy only after medical treatment failure.

► HODGKIN'S DISEASE STAGING

Because of the favorable success of salvage chemotherapy in the treatment of Hodgkin's lymphoma, the need for determining whether disease is present across the diaphragm by means of laparotomy and splenectomy has sharply declined. Treatment with salvage chemotherapy after local radiation failure still carries a highly favorable outcome in most cases. Therefore, splenectomy for staging Hodgkin's disease is now rarely performed.

► OVERWHELMING POSTSPLENECTOMY SEPSIS

Asplenic individuals are at greater risk for developing fulminant bacteremia because of decreased opsonic activity, decreased levels of IgM, and decreased clearance of bacteria from the blood after splenectomy. As a rule, children are at greater risk for developing sepsis than adults, and fatal sepsis is more common after splenectomy for hematologic disorders than after trauma. The risk of sepsis is higher in the first postoperative year, and, for adults, each subsequent year carries approximately a 1% chance of developing sepsis. The clinical picture of OPSS is the onset of high fever followed by circulatory collapse from septic shock. Disseminated intravascular coagulation often occurs. The offending pathogens are the encapsulated bacteria *Streptococcus pneumoniae*, *Haemophilus influenzae*, and *Neisseria meningitidis*.

Concern regarding OPSS has spurred efforts to perform partial splenectomy or splenorrhaphy in trauma to preserve splenic function. Vaccination against pneumococcal sepsis with the pneumococcal polyvalent polysaccharide vaccine should be administered to all surgically and functionally asplenic patients.

Key Points

1. ITP, hypersplenism, and specific hemolytic anemias are disease states for which splenectomy may be indicated.

2. Splenectomy for staging Hodgkin's disease is rarely performed anymore because of the success of salvage chemotherapy.

3. The risk of OPSS is greater in children than adults. High fever and septic shock are often accompanied by DIC.

4. *Streptococcus pneumoniae*, *Haemophilus influenzae*, and *Neisseria meningitidis* are encapsulated organisms responsible for causing OPSS.

5. Vaccination against pneumococcal sepsis should be administered to all surgically and functionally asplenic patients.

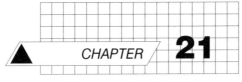

CHAPTER 21

Thyroid Gland

*S*urgical thyroid disease encompasses those conditions in which partial or complete removal of the thyroid gland is required due to goiter and hyperthyroid conditions unresponsive to medical management and to benign and malignant neoplastic disease.

▶ ANATOMY AND PHYSIOLOGY

The thyroid gland is derived embryologically from an evagination of the floor of the pharynx at the base of the tongue. The developing thyroid descends along a midline course to its final position as a bilobed gland overlying the lower half of the thyroid cartilage. The two lateral lobes of the fully developed gland are connected by a median isthmus. In 75% of individuals, the distal thyroglossal remnant extends superiorly from the isthmus and is called the pyramidal lobe. Arterial blood is supplied via the paired superior and inferior thyroid arteries, and venous drainage is via the paired superior, middle, and inferior thyroid veins (Fig. 21-1).

Of key importance to the surgeon is anatomic knowledge of the recurrent laryngeal nerve. Bilateral vagus nerves descend from the neck into the chest. The right vagus branches into the right recurrent laryngeal nerve, which loops under the right subclavian artery from anterior to posterior and ascends superiorly in the right tracheoesophageal groove. The left vagus branches into the left recurrent laryngeal nerve, which loops in a similar anterior to posterior fashion around the arch of the aorta and ascends along the left tracheoesophageal groove. The recurrent laryngeal nerves travel posteromedial to their respective thyroid lobes and enter the larynx via the cricothyroid membrane to innervate the abductor muscles of the true vocal cords. Injury during thyroidectomy results in ipsilateral vocal cord paralysis and subsequent hoarseness (Fig. 21-2).

Due to aberrant migration of the developing thyroid gland, several anatomic variances can be seen. Complete failure of migration from the base of the

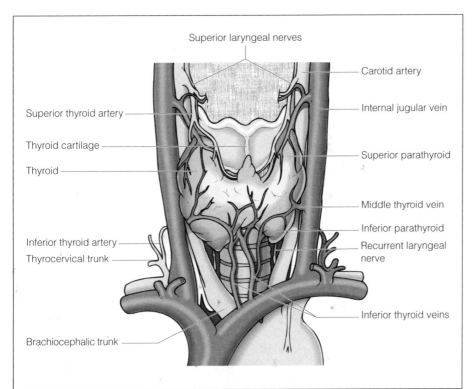

Figure 21-1 Anatomy of the thyroid gland.

Superior laryngeal nerves

Carotid artery

Superior thyroid artery

Internal jugular vein

Thyroid cartilage

Superior parathyroid

Thyroid

Middle thyroid vein

Inferior parathyroid

Inferior thyroid artery

Recurrent laryngeal nerve

Thyrocervical trunk

Inferior thyroid veins

Brachiocephalic trunk

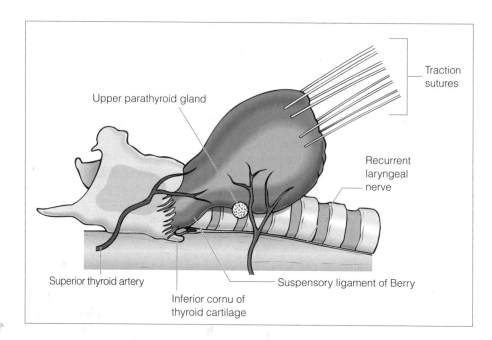

Figure 21-2 Course of the recurrent laryngeal nerve.

tongue results in a **lingual thyroid**. The entire mass of thyroid tissue is located in the posterior tongue, and airway obstruction may result if goiter develops. Incomplete migration can result in thyroid tissue being found anywhere between the base of the tongue and the root of the neck. Lastly, thyroid tissue may migrate beyond the level of the thyroid cartilage into the substernal region, where occasionally a substernal goiter develops.

Persistence of the thyroglossal duct results in a **thyroglossal cyst** or **fistula**. Thyroglossal cysts are most commonly seen in children and present as a single painless lump in the midline that moves with swallowing. Surgical excision of the cyst is corrective. Thyroglossal duct fistulae present as midline sinus tracts. As the fistula is an embryological remnant, it ascends superiorly through the middle of the hyoid bone, often to its origin at the base of the tongue. Surgical excision of the fistula requires resection of the middle portion of the hyoid bone (Fig. 21-3).

The thyroid gland determines the metabolic pace of the body. Increased levels of thyroid hormone and loss of the normal negative feedback mechanism result in hyperthyroidism. The main etiologies of hyperthyroidism are (a) diffuse toxic goiter (Graves' disease), (b) toxic multinodular goiter (Plummer's disease), and (c) toxic adenoma. Surgical treatment of these disorders involves either excision of localized diseased tissue, as in the case of adenoma, or complete excision of the majority of the gland, as in Graves' disease or toxic multinodular goiter.

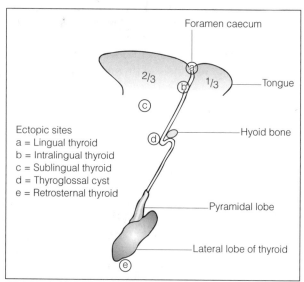

Figure 21-3 Migration of the thyroid via the thyroglossal duct and possible ectopic sites of development and duct remnants.

▶ GRAVES' DISEASE

The most common cause of hyperthyroidism in the United States and Europe is Graves' disease. This autoimmune disorder is caused by thyroid-stimulating immunoglobulins that target the thyroid-stimulating hormone (TSH) receptor of the thyroid gland. The hyperstimulated gland releases excessive amounts of hormone, resulting in the classic clinical picture of goiter, exophthalmos, pretibial myxedema, and the signs and symptoms of hyperthyroidism. The exact pathogenesis remains unclear; however, evidence of a genetic component exists in many cases. Families with Graves' disease exhibit an overall increased incidence of thyroid disorders and increased levels of circulating antithyroid antibodies. Individuals and families with Graves' disease also have higher incidences of other autoimmune disorders such as insulin-dependent diabetes mellitus, rheumatoid arthritis, and Addison's disease.

History

The typical presentation of hyperthyroidism involves complaints of unexplained nervousness and sweating, heat intolerance, weight loss, palpitations, an enlarging neck mass, and ocular prominence. As patients will present at different stages of disease, the subtle findings of early disease differ dramatically from the florid exophthalmos, dyspnea, and agitation of more advanced cases.

Physical Examination

Patients are generally agitated, irritable, or nervous. The enlarged gland is palpable and often visibly apparent. Due to increased vascularity, a thrill may be felt or a bruit auscultated over the enlarged lobes.

The most notable and dramatic finding is exophthalmos, caused by edema of the retrobulbar fat pad forcing the globe anteriorly. Increased sympathetic tone secondary to excess thyroid hormone causes eyelid retraction, leading to the pronounced Graves' "stare."

Skin exam reveals myxedema, a raised plaque-like skin change seen typically in a pretibial distribution. Cardiac examination demonstrates sinus tachycardia, hyperdynamism, systolic flow murmurs, and occasionally atrial fibrillation.

Diagnostic Evaluation

Thyroid function tests will yield the information necessary for making the diagnosis of Graves' disease. T3 and T4 levels are elevated due to gland hyperstimulation and the TSH level is low due to the negative feedback exerted by circulating thyroid hormones. If T3 and T4 levels are within normal limits, radioactive iodide uptake testing (RAIU) will show increased uptake secondary to increased glandular activity.

Thyrotropin-releasing hormone (TRH) testing will show a negative response in Graves' disease. TSH will not rise in response to IV infusion of TRH since pituitary secretion has been inhibited by negative feedback.

Differential Diagnosis

Thyroiditis, factitious hyperthyroidism, anxiety disorder.

Treatment

Hyperthyroidism of Graves' disease is treated by either:

1. Antithyroid medication to reduce glandular hormone secretion;
2. Radioiodine ablation to reduce the functional glandular mass; or
3. Surgical excision.

The appropriate treatment choice is determined by considerations such as pregnancy status, surgical risk, and treatment side effects.

Antithyroid Medication

The goal of antithyroid medication is to return the patient to a euthyroid state. Two thiocarbamide medications, propylthiouracil (PTU) and methimazole (Tapazole), inhibit thyroid hormone synthesis. Additionally, propylthiouracil inhibits peripheral conversion of T4 to T3. Despite the ability of antithyroid medications to control the signs and symptoms of hyperthyroidism, there is a high recurrence rate. Hence, such medications are used for long-term treatment of patients expected to undergo remission as indicated by mild laboratory abnormalities and a small goiter.

Adjunctive drug therapy includes beta-blockers to control the signs and symptoms of thyrotoxicosis. Propranolol is used to dampen the increased sympathetic tone brought on by circulating thyroid hormones. Iodide is used to inhibit thyroid hormone release directly and treat patients with severe disease rapidly. Iodine may also be used preoperatively before elective thyroidectomy to reduce glandular vascularity.

Radioactive Iodine Therapy

Radioactive ablation of the thyroid with I^{131} is simple and effective. The goal of therapy is to reduce the functional mass of thyroid tissue to achieve a euthyroid level of secretion. However, the final result is often complete glandular ablation with subsequent permanent hypothyroidism requiring life-long thyroid hormone replacement. Radioactive iodine therapy is useful for most patients, except pregnant women and newborns.

Subtotal Thyroidectomy

Surgical intervention is appropriate for patients with contraindications to radioactive iodine therapy and for patients unable to tolerate or who are unresponsive to antithyroid medications. Children and young adults comprise the majority of such patients. As with radioiodine therapy, the goal of surgical treatment is to reduce the mass of thyroid tissue to a level where eu-thyroid levels of hormone are secreted by residual tissue. Despite the low operative risk of the proce-dure, significant complications can include recur-rent laryngeal nerve injury with vocal cord paralysis, permanent hypothyroidism, and surgical hypopara-thyroidism. Despite undergoing surgery, recurrent hy-perthyroidism occurs in approximately 5% of patients.

The operation is performed through a curvilinear "necklace" incision extending to the sternocleidomas-toid muscles bilaterally. Of key importance is to avoid injury to the recurrent laryngeal nerves, parathyroid glands, and the external branches of the superior la-ryngeal nerves.

Follow-Up

After treatment, thyroid function tests should be mea-sured to ensure the patient is euthyroid. This is impor-tant since up to 50% of patients may develop postop-erative hypothyroidism and require thyroid hormone replacement therapy.

▶ THYROID CANCER

Thyroid cancers are relatively uncommon since they account for only about 1% of all malignancies. The four thyroid cancer types are papillary, follicular, medul-lary, and anaplastic. The tumor types differ in histo-logic appearance, malignant behavior, and treatment response. Indolent papillary cancer carries a favorable 80% ten-year survival rate, while undifferentiated ana-plastic cancer is invariably fatal. Anaplastic thyroid cancer is one of the most lethal cancers known, with an average life expectancy of 5 months from the time of diagnosis. Follicular and medullary cancers occupy the middle ground. Depending on the tumor type, surgical therapy has variable success.

Pathogenesis

Although the etiology of most thyroid cancer is un-known, cancer of the thyroid has been experimentally induced by exposure to radiation, goitrogenic medica-tions, and iodide deficiency. Knowledge of radiation-induced carcinogenesis evolved from experience with the use of external beam radiation as medical therapy earlier this century. It was noted that a significant number of children irradiated for the treatment of acne, enlarged tonsils, or hemangiomas subsequently developed thyroid cancer, usually of papillary type. A direct dose-response relationship was identified, showing that the incidence of malignancy was propor-tional to the radiation dose received. Eventually it was discovered that ionizing radiation exerts a dual carci-nogenic role: the disruption of cellular DNA and the inducement of chronic TSH stimulation of the thyroid gland by damaging the capacity to produce thyroid hormone necessary for negative feedback.

History

Patients usually present for surgical evaluation after an asymptomatic painless **thyroid nodule** is discov-ered on routine physical exam. A systemic work-up for a newly diagnosed thyroid nodule is necessary to de-termine the biologic nature of the nodule and to rule out cancer. Nodules may present at any age, but younger patients are more likely to have a malignant nodule than are older patients. Important historical information includes the duration of nodule existence, rate of enlargement, presence of voice changes, dys-phagia, prior radiation exposure from medical or mil-itary sources, radioiodine therapy in childhood, a fam-ily history of medullary cancer, and a history of iodide deficiency suggested by residence in a geographic area of endemic goiter.

Physical Examination

Physical findings may range from a single discrete nodule in a single lobe, to large bulky disease with evidence of distant metastasis. Generally, carcinomas are nontender on palpation; however, pain may arise after hemorrhage into a necrotic tumor or by compres-sion of local structures. Hoarseness is often a sign of malignancy, indicating invasion of the recurrent la-ryngeal nerve. An enlarging fixed nodule with associ-ated adenopathy and symptoms of dysphagia also sug-gests malignancy.

Differential Diagnosis

The differential diagnosis of a thyroid nodule includes:

▲ follicular adenoma
▲ multinodular goiter
▲ colloid nodule
▲ hashimoto's thyroiditis
▲ thyroid cyst
▲ thyroid lymphoma
▲ papillary thyroid cancer
▲ follicular thyroid cancer
▲ medullary thyroid cancer
▲ anaplastic thyroid cancer
▲ metastatic cancer
▲ parathyroid mass

Diagnostic Evaluation

The goal of the preoperative evaluation of a thyroid nodule is to obtain a diagnosis so that appropriate treatment, either medical or surgical, can be administered. Standard thyroid function tests reveal the functional status of the gland and are rarely abnormal in patients with thyroid cancer.

The single most important diagnostic study is percutaneous fine-needle aspiration since it provides a tissue diagnosis. Other useful studies include radionuclide thyroid scanning, which demonstrates the functional status of a nodule by showing whether a nodule is "hot" or "cold." A hot functioning nodule takes up high levels of radioactive iodide tracer and is almost always benign. A cold nodule indicates low uptake and minimal function. Cold nodules are suspicious for cancer and should be surgically removed. Thyroid ultrasound is used to determine whether a nodule is solid or cystic, to assess nodule size, or to identify impalpable nodules. Solid nodules are more likely to be cancerous than are cystic lesions. For patients suspected of having medullary cancer based on family history, serum calcitonin levels should be checked after a calcium-pentagastrin infusion test. An elevated calcitonin level defines a positive result.

Treatment

Papillary

Usually associated with exposure to ionizing radiation, papillary thyroid cancer is often multicentric and bilateral, spreading slowly via lymphatic channels to lymph nodes and by direct extension into surrounding structures. Only 5% of patients with papillary cancer present with distant metastases. For tumors less than 1.5 cm and for disease confined clinically to one lobe, thyroid lobectomy is generally performed. However, due to the multicentric and often bilateral nature of the disease, some surgeons advocate total thyroidectomy since a more extensive operation is associated with lower rates of recurrence and better long-term survival.

Follicular

Found more commonly in iodide-deficient regions, follicular thyroid cancer usually presents as a solitary thyroid mass. Tumors invade vascular structures, and metastasis is by hematologic spread to brain, bone, lungs, and liver. Total thyroidectomy is indicated.

Medullary

Typically seen as part of multiple endocrine neoplasia disease, medullary thyroid cancer is usually multicentric and bilateral, with early metastasis to cervical lymph nodes. Total thyroidectomy is performed with additional neck dissection if lymph node metastases are present.

Anaplastic

A lethal cancer seen more frequently in regions with endemic goiter, anaplastic thyroid cancers usually present as rapidly enlarging neck masses. Extremely aggressive tumor invasion into vital neck structures may cause dysphagia and dyspnea. Tracheal invasion is common and tracheostomy may be required to maintain airway patency. Such invasiveness usually precludes surgical resection, and attempts at palliation with radiation therapy and chemotherapy are limited.

▶ KEY POINTS

1. The thyroid gland is derived from an evagination at the base of the tongue followed by migration into the neck via the thyroglossal duct. Failure of thyroid migration results in a lingual thyroid, while persistence of the thyroglossal duct results in a thyroglossal cyst or fistula.

2. The recurrent laryngeal nerve may be damaged during surgery, causing ipsilateral vocal cord paralysis and hoarseness.

3. Graves' disease, toxic multinodular goiter, and toxic adenoma are the main etiologies of hyperthyroidism.

4. Graves' disease is an autoimmune disorder caused by thyroid-stimulating immunoglobulins that target TSH receptors of the thyroid gland.

5. T3 and T4 levels are elevated in Graves' disease while the TSH level is low due to negative feedback.

6. Management of Graves' disease includes antithyroid medications, radioiodine ablation, or surgical excision.

7. Complications of subtotal thyroidectomy include recurrent laryngeal nerve injury, permanent hypothyroidism, and surgical hypoparathyroidism.

8. The four types of thyroid cancer in order of increasing malignancy are papillary, follicular, medullary, and anaplastic.

9. Fine-needle aspiration is the most important diagnostic study for evaluation of a thyroid nodule.

10. Medullary cancer patients have an elevated calcitonin level on calcium-pentagastrin testing.

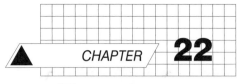

CHAPTER 22

Trauma

*7*raumatic injury and death are a major problem in the United States, where approximately 60 million injuries occur annually. Trauma is the leading cause of death in the first four decades of life, and the third leading cause of overall death, trailing only cancer and coronary artery disease. Although approximately 150,000 traumatic deaths occur annually, the rate of disability from trauma is three times greater than mortality. Therefore, issues relating to trauma care are of importance to all medical and surgical specialists, from the trauma surgeon to the rehabilitation specialist.

Death due to trauma has been shown to occur in a trimodal distribution, during three identifiable time periods. The first peak of death occurs within seconds to minutes of injury. Lethal injury to the body's vital anatomic structures leads to rapid death unless immediate advanced intervention is performed. The second peak of death occurs within minutes to several hours after the injury. Death during this second period is usually due to progressive neurologic, cardiovascular, or pulmonary compromise. It is during this intermediate period that patients have the greatest chance of salvage and toward which organized trauma care is focused. Rapid resuscitation coupled with the identification and treatment of both potentially lethal injuries is the goal. The final third peak of death occurs several days to weeks after initial injury, usually secondary to sepsis and multiorgan system failure.

This chapter will discuss trauma management during the above-mentioned second period. Specifically, the steps of the initial assessment performed when the trauma patient arrives at the hospital emergency room, the primary survey of the patient (ABCs), resuscitation, the secondary survey (head-to-toe), and the institution of definitive care will be examined.

▶ PRIMARY SURVEY

The focus of the primary survey is to identify immediately life-threatening conditions and prevent death. Without a patent airway, adequate gas exchange, or sufficient intravascular volume, any patient will die. Therefore, a simple mnemonic is used to direct the primary survey:

Airway with cervical spine control

Breathing and ventilation

Circulation and hemorrhage control

Disability and neurologic assessment

Exposure to enable examination

(A) The airway is immediately inspected to ensure that patency and any causes of airway obstruction are identified (foreign body, facial fracture, tracheal/laryngeal disruption, cervical spine injury). Cervical spine control must be maintained at all times since patients with multitrauma must be assumed to have cervical spine injury until cleared radiographically. The chin thrust and jaw lift are methods of initially establishing airway patency while simultaneously protecting the cervical spine.

(B) Once airway patency is established, the patient's ability to breathe must be assessed. Normal function of the lungs, chest wall, and diaphragm is necessary for ventilation and gas exchange to occur. Auscultation, visual inspection, and palpation of the chest may indicate the presence of a tension pneumothorax, open pneumothorax, massive hemothorax, or flail chest segment with underlying pulmonary contusion. Needle decompression, chest tube placement, or endotracheal intubation may be required to ensure adequate ventilation.

(C) Hypotension secondary to hemorrhage can result from both penetrating and blunt trauma. External hemorrhage can usually be identified and controlled by direct manual pressure. Tourniquets should be avoided since they cause distal ischemia. Internal hemorrhage is more difficult to identify. Therefore, hypotension without signs of external hemorrhage must be assumed to be due to intra-abdominal or intrathoracic injury, or from fractures of the pelvis or long bones. The hypovolemic hypotensive patient will usually exhibit a diminished level of consciousness as cerebral blood flow is reduced, the pulse will be rapid and thready, and the skin will be pale and clammy.

(D) Traumatic injuries may cause damage to the central and peripheral nervous system. Spinal cord injuries are most commonly seen in the cervical and lumbar regions. The thoracic spine is less prone to injury due to the rigidity of the bony thorax. Complete spinal cord injury affects all neurologic function below a specific level of the cord. Incomplete spinal cord injury exhibits sacral sparing and may involve (a) the central portion of the cord as in the central cord syndrome, (b) a single side of the cord as in Brown-Séquard syndrome, or (c) the anterior portion of the cord as in anterior cord syndrome. A rapid assessment of disability and neurologic function is vital so that drug therapy and physical maneuvers can be initiated to prevent further neurologic injury.

(E) Exposure of the trauma patient is important so that the entire body can be examined and injuries diagnosed. Complete exposure entails the removal of all clothing from the patient so that a thorough examination can be performed, allowing for identification of entry and exit wounds, extremity deformities, contusions, or lacerations.

▶ RESUSCITATION

The resuscitation phase of trauma management occurs almost simultaneously with the initial survey since once a life-threatening condition is identified, the appropriate management is initiated. Airway control and ventilation are the first priorities for any trauma patient.

Airway control in the conscious patient can be achieved with an easily inserted nasopharyngeal trumpet, whereas an oropharyngeal airway is utilized in the unconscious patient. Definitive control of the airway and enhanced ability to ventilate and oxygenate the patient are achieved with endotracheal intubation. Tube placement may be via the nasal or oral route. Nasotracheal intubation is a useful technique for patients with cervical spine injuries; however, it is contraindicated when midface or basilar skull fractures are suspected. When the trachea is unable to be intubated, a surgical airway is indicated. Jet insufflation of the airway after needle cricothyroidotomy can adequately oxygenate patients for 30 to 45 minutes. Surgical cricothyroidotomy with the insertion of a tracheostomy or endotracheal tube allows prolonged ventilation and oxygenation.

Injuries to the chest may acutely impair the ability to provide adequate ventilation. The chest must be examined for evidence of tension pneumothorax, open pneumothorax, hemothorax, and flail chest. The clinical picture of hypotension, tachycardia, tracheal deviation, neck vein distention, and diminished unilateral breath sounds suggests the diagnosis of tension pneumothorax. Immediate decompression by the insertion of a needle catheter into the second intercostal space in the midclavicular line is indicated, followed by definitive treatment with chest tube insertion into the fifth intercostal space at the anterior axillary line just lateral to the nipple. Open pneumothorax requires closure of the chest wall defect, hemothorax requires the insertion of a large caliber chest tube for drainage of blood, and most patients with flail chest secondary to multiple rib fractures have underlying pulmonary contusion and may require eventual intubation to prevent hypoxia.

Hemorrhage leading to hypovolemic shock is the most common cause of postinjury death in the trauma patient. Rapid fluid resuscitation and hemorrhage control are the keys to restoring adequate circulating blood volume. The fluid status of patients can be quickly evaluated by assessing their hemodynamics (hypotension and tachycardia), by their level of consciousness (adequacy of cerebral perfusion), by the color of their skin (pale skin indicates significant exsanguination), and by the presence and character of the pulse (absent central pulses indicate profound hypovolemic shock). All sources of external hemorrhage must be identified and treated by the application of direct pressure. Indiscriminate hemostat usage should be avoided as well since it may crush and damage surrounding neurovascular structures. Sources of internal hemorrhage are usually hidden and are suspected by unstable hemodynamics. Internal bleeding may occur in the thorax due to cardiovascular or pulmonary injury, in the abdomen from splenic or liver lacerations, or into the soft tissues surrounding femur or pelvic fractures.

Fluid resuscitation of the hypovolemic hypotensive patient requires the establishment of adequate intravenous access. Two large bore intravenous catheters (14 gauge) should be placed in upper extremity veins and rapid infusion of a balanced salt solution (LR or NS) initiated. If the pattern of injury allows, central access via the femoral vein approach using larger diameter catheters maximizes the rate of fluid administration. If percutaneous access is unsuccessful, a cutdown of the greater saphenous vein at the anteromedial ankle is required. After intravenous access is established, bolus infusion of crystalloid solution should be replaced with O-negative or type-specific blood once it becomes available.

▶ TRAUMA ROENTGENOGRAMS

For patients with blunt trauma (automobile crashes, falls), three standard radiographic studies are required to assess the neck, chest, and pelvis: cross-table lateral cervical spine, anteroposterior chest, and anteroposterior pelvis. Obtaining these three x-rays early in the resuscitation process allows potentially neurologically disabling cervical spine injuries, life-threatening chest wall and cardiopulmonary injuries, and pelvic injuries to be identified and immediately treated. For patients with penetrating trauma (gunshots, stabbings, impalings), an anteroposterior chest film and other films pertaining to the site of injury should be obtained.

▶ SECONDARY SURVEY

The secondary survey begins after the airway, breathing, and circulation have been assessed and resuscitation has been initiated. This secondary survey is a head-to-toe evaluation of the body during which additional areas of injury are identified. A meticulous examination during this phase of the trauma evaluation minimizes the chance of missing an important finding.

The final phase of acute trauma care is the institution of definitive treatment. This may entail simple wound care in the emergency room for minor injuries or, if the injuries warrant, transportation to the operating room for surgical treatment.

Key Points

1. Trauma is the leading cause of death in the first four decades of life.

2. Trauma is the third leading cause of death overall, after cancer and heart disease.

3. Traumatic death occurs in a trimodal distribution.

4. Trauma care involves the primary survey, resuscitation, secondary survey, and definitive care.

5. The primary survey identifies immediately life-threatening injuries involving the airway, breathing, and circulation (ABC).

6. Resuscitation involves airway control and ventilation, and fluid infusion after intravenous access is obtained.

7. The secondary survey is a head-to-toe examination to identify additional areas of injury.

8. Standard roentgenograms required for trauma include: lateral cervical spine, AP chest, AP pelvis.

▶ OPHTHALMIC TRAUMA

More than 1 million cases of ophthalmic trauma after penetrating or blunt injury are reported annually in the United States. Prompt and appropriate care of many ophthalmic injuries may prevent much visual disability.

Chemical Burns

Chemical burns to the eye represent an ophthalmologic emergency. If treatment is not begun immediately, irreversible damage may occur. Alkaline substances (i.e., household cleaners, fertilizers, and pesticides) cause the most severe damage, but acids may cause significant ocular morbidity as well.

Treatment

A detailed history is not required before beginning copious irrigation with any available water source for at least 15 to 20 minutes. After initial irrigation, visual acuity and pH should be measured. If the pH has not returned to the normal value of 7.5, irrigation should be continued. Prompt ophthalmologic referral should be obtained in all cases of acid or alkali burns and for patients with decreased visual acuity, severe conjunctival swelling, or corneal clouding. All other patients should see an ophthalmologist within 24 hours.

Key Points

1. Chemical burns to the eye are a true ophthalmologic emergency.

2. Detailed history is not necessary.

3. Treatment consists of a copious irrigation followed by prompt referral to an ophthalmologist.

Superficial Foreign Bodies

Foreign bodies that have an impact on the surface of the cornea or conjunctiva represent approximately 25% of all ocular injuries.

History

An accurate history often provides the diagnosis and should be used to judge the risk of intraocular foreign body (see below). Symptoms range from mild ocular irritation to severe pain. If symptoms began gradually rather than suddenly, one must consider other etiologies such as infectious keratitis.

Diagnostic Evaluation

Careful inspection of the cornea and conjuctiva using bright light and magnification will often reveal the foreign body.

Treatment

Always measure visual acuity before any attempt at foreign body removal. Superficial foreign bodies can usually be removed using topical anesthesia and a cotton swab. After the foreign body is removed, Wood's lamp examination with fluorescein should be performed to ascertain the size of any residual corneal epithelial defect. Eversion of the upper eyelid should be carried out to look for residual foreign material under the lids. Topical antibiotics should be instilled, and patients should be followed daily until all fluorescein staining resolves. Ophthalmologic referral is indicated when a foreign body cannot safely be removed or for any patient with a large corneal epithelial defect.

Key Points

1. An accurate history should provide the clue to a diagnosis of conjunctival or corneal foreign body.

2. Superficial foreign bodies may be removed under topical anesthesia.

3. Any resulting corneal abrasion requires appropriate treatment and follow-up.

Blunt or Penetrating Injury

Blunt or penetrating trauma to the eye represents a leading cause of vision loss in young people. Blunt trauma most often causes ocular contusion or damage to the surrounding orbit. Penetrating trauma causes corneal or scleral laceration (a ruptured globe) and represents an ophthalmologic emergency requiring early intervention and repair. The possibility of a retained intraocular foreign body should always be considered (see below). A high degree of suspicion must be maintained in all cases of head and facial trauma to avoid missing significant ocular or orbital injury.

History

History should include the mechanism of injury, the force of impact, the likelihood of a retained foreign body, and any associated ocular or visual complaints.

Diagnostic Evaluation

Eyelid integrity, ocular motility, and pupillary reaction should be tested. Using a pen light, conjunctival swelling or hemorrhage, corneal or scleral laceration, or hyphema (blood behind the cornea obscuring details of the underlying iris or pupil) should be noted. Pain and decreased vision with a history of trauma should always lead one to suspect perforation of the globe. Severe subconjunctival hemorrhage, a shallow anterior chamber or space between the cornea and iris, hyphema, and limitation of extraocular motility are often, but not invariably, present. Radiologic studies including computed tomography of the head and orbits should be obtained in cases of suspected blow-out fracture or to rule out a retained intraocular foreign body (see below).

Treatment

If the eye is lacerated or the pupil or iris is not visible, a shield should be placed over the eye, and the patient

---

TABLE 22-1

Management of Ophthalmic Trauma

Treat on-site and refer immediately
  Acid or alkali burn
  Unremovable corneal or conjunctival foreign body
Refer immediately
  Severe pain
  Subnormal visual acuity
  Irregular pupil
  Deformed globe
  Corneal or scleral laceration
  Corneal clouding
  Severe lid swelling
  Severe conjunctival chemosis
  Proptosis
  Hyphema
  Absent red reflex
  Suspected intraocular foreign body (history of being struck by high-speed missile)
  Eyelid laceration that is deep, large, avulsed, exposes fat, or extends through lid margin or lacrimal drainage apparatus

Refer within 24 hours
  Pain
  Photophobia
  Diplopia
  Foreign-body sensation but no visible foreign body or corneal abrasion
  Large corneal abrasion
  Moderate eyelid or conjunctival chemosis but normal visual acuity
  Suspected contusion of globe
  Suspected orbital wall fracture

Refer within 48 hours
  Mild contusion injury to orbital soft tissues

---

should be referred immediately to an ophthalmologist. Eyelid lacerations that involve the lid margin or lacrimal apparatus require meticulous repair to avoid severe functional and cosmetic morbidity. If the eyelid margin and inner one sixth of the eyelid are not damaged, the wound may be closed with fine sutures. If the eyelid margin is lacerated, accurate realignment of the lid margin must be ensured before wound closure. Disruption of the inner one sixth of the eyelid requires intubation of the lacrimal drainage system with stent placement before surgical repair and should be carried out by an ophthalmologist or other appropriately trained physician. Ophthalmologic referral after trauma is determined by ocular symptoms and findings, as set forth in Table 22-1.

Key Points

1. Given a history of severe trauma, a ruptured globe should be presumed to exist.

2. No attempt should be made to examine a ruptured globe in the emergency room setting, and the eye should be shielded while awaiting evaluation by an ophthalmologist.

3. Simple eyelid lacerations may be repaired once disruption of the lid margin and lacrimal apparatus is excluded.

Intraocular Foreign Bodies

A high-speed missile may penetrate the cornea or sclera while causing minimal symptoms or physical findings. Foreign body composition is important because certain metals such as iron, steel, and copper will produce a severe inflammatory reaction if left in the eye, whereas other materials such as glass, lead, and stone are relatively inert and may not require surgical removal. Retained vegetable matter is especially dangerous and may cause a severe purulent endophthalmitis. A retained foreign body should be suspected in all cases of perforating injuries of the eye or whenever the history suggests high-risk activities such as drilling, sawing, or hammering.

History

One should inquire about high-risk activities, a sensation of sudden impact on the eyelids or eye, and any complaint of pain or decreased vision.

Physical Examination

Visual acuity should always be recorded before any manipulation of the eye or eyelids. Inspection may reveal an entry wound, although this may be quite subtle and easily overlooked. One should specifically look for a hyphema, pupillary distortion, or any alteration of the red reflex on funduscopic examination.

Diagnostic Evaluation

Accurate localization may require soft tissue roentgenograms, orbital ultrasound, or computed tomography. Magnetic resonance imaging is contraindicated in all cases of suspected intraocular foreign body.

Treatment

If the history strongly suggests the possibility of a retained foreign body, urgent ophthalmologic referral is indicated even in the absence of physical findings. Prompt surgical removal of intraocular debris is usually indicated to avoid the toxic effect of metallic foreign bodies on intraocular tissue and to avoid secondary intraocular infection from retained organic material.

Key Points

1. An accurate history is important.

2. Refer immediately any high-speed missile injury to the eye, even in the absence of physical findings.

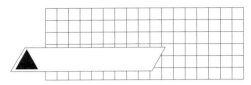

References

Anderson JE. Grant's atlas of anatomy. 8th ed. Baltimore: Williams & Wilkins, 1983.

Cameron JL. Current surgical therapy. 5th ed. St. Louis: Mosby, 1995.

Clemente CD. Anatomy. 3rd ed. Baltimore: Urban and Schwarzenberg, 1987.

Fitzpatrick TB. Color atlas and synopsis of clinical dermatology. 2nd ed. New York: McGraw-Hill, 1992.

Greenfield L. Surgery: scientific principles and practice. Philadelphia: J.B. Lippincott, 1993.

Jarrell B. Surgery: National Medical Series (NMS). New York: Wiley Medical, 1986.

Lawrence PF. Essentials of general surgery. Baltimore: Williams and Wilkins, 1988.

Morris P, Malt R. Oxford textbook of surgery. Oxford: Oxford University Press, 1994.

Newell FW. Ophthalmology: principles and concepts. 7th ed. St. Louis: Mosby-Year Book, 1992.

Osteen RT, ed. Cancer manual of the American Cancer Society. 8th ed. Boston: 1990.

Sabiston DC Jr. Textbook of surgery. 14th ed. Philadelphia: WB Saunders, 1991.

Sadler TW. Langman's medical embryology. 6th ed. Baltimore: Williams & Wilkins, 1990.

Schwartz SI, Shires GT, Spencer FC. Principles of surgery. 6th ed. New York: McGraw-Hill, 1995.

Simmons R, Steed D. Basic science review for surgeons. Philadelphia: WB Saunders, 1992.

Trobe JD. The Physician's guide to eye care. San Francisco: American Academy of Ophthalmology, 1993.

Vaughn DG, Asbury T, Riordan-Eva P. General ophthalmology. 13th ed. Norwalk, CT: Appleton & Lange, 1992.

Veith FJ, Hobson RW, Williams RA, Wilson SE. Vascular surgery. 2nd ed. New York: McGraw-Hill, 1994.

Way L. Current surgical diagnosis & treatment. 9th ed. Norwalk, CT: Appleton & Lange, 1991.

Index